FOODS THAT FIGHT
FIBROMYALGIA

Nutrient-Packed Meals That INCREASE ENERGY, EASE PAIN, and Move You Towards RECOVERY

DEIRDRE RAWLINGS, PH.D., N.D.

WITH FOREWORD BY **JACOB TEITELBAUM, M.D.**

FAIR WINDS
PRESS

First published in the USA in 2012 by
Fair Winds Press, a member of
Quarto Publishing Group USA Inc.
100 Cummings Center
Suite 406-L
Beverly, MA 01915-6101
www.fairwindspress.com

ISBN: 978-1-59233-539-8

Digital edition published in 2012
eISBN: 978-1-61058-632-0

Library of Congress Cataloging-in-Publication Data available

Book design: Visible Logic
Photography: Glenn Scott Photography
Food stylist: Catrine Kelty

Printed and bound in USA

An earlier edition of this book was published under the title *Food that Helps Win the
Battle Against Fibromyalgia*.

*The information in this book is for educational purposes only. It is not intended to replace
the advice of a physician or medical practitioner. Please see your health care provider before
beginning any new health program.*

This book is dedicated to Jonathan, whose love, support,
and generous spirit were guiding energies behind this book.

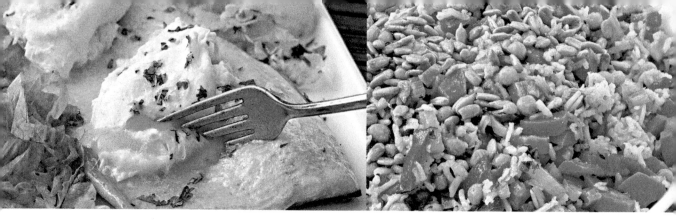

CONTENTS

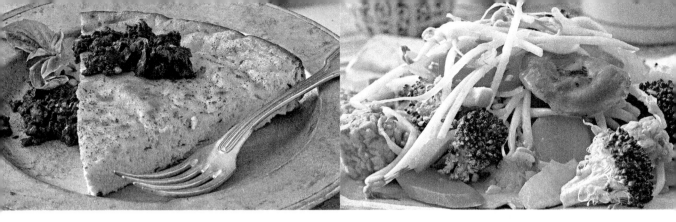

FOREWORD

Cases of fibromyalgia and its painful cousin, chronic fatigue syndrome (CFS), are increasing in epidemic proportions—incidence rates have swelled by 400 to 1,000 percent in the last decade alone. As Deirdre Rawlings notes in this excellent book, these syndromes represent an energy crisis in our body. In fact, they are illnesses of modern life, caused by poor nutrition, poor sleep, hormonal deficiencies, and various sources of stress (infections, injuries, toxic chemicals, toxic bosses). Simply put, anything that causes you to spend more energy than you can make will result in an energy crisis. When this occurs, the area of the brain that uses the most energy for its size (the hypothalamus) is the first to malfunction—like blowing a fuse. This center controls sleep, hormones, temperature, blood flow, blood pressure, and sweating, and its malfunction produces many of the symptoms associated with fibromyalgia. In addition, if your muscles do not have enough energy, they get stuck in a shortened position and you feel pain. The chronic pain trigger then causes changes in your brain that amplify the pain (called central sensitization). The good news is that this is all very treatable.

Ready to Get Well?

Four key areas need to be treated to switch back on your "circuit breaker" and resolve your fatigue and pain. Think SHIN.

SLEEP. Because the hypothalamic circuit breaker that normally controls sleep is offline, most patients need a mix of natural and prescription sleep treatments. To get well and feel pain free, it is critical that you use appropriate and effective sleep treatments to get eight to nine hours of sleep every night.

HORMONAL DEFICIENCIES. The hypothalamus is the main control center, via the pituitary, for most of the glands in the body. Most of the normal ranges for our blood tests were not developed in the context of hypothalamic suppression or these syndromes. Because of this (and for a number of other reasons), it is usually necessary to treat with natural thyroid, adrenal, ovarian, and testicular hormones. These hormones have been found to be fairly safe, when used in low doses.

INFECTIONS. Many studies have shown immune system dysfunction in people with fibromyalgia, which can result in many unusual infections. These include viral infections, parasites and other bowel infections, and most importantly fungal/candida infections. The nutritional therapies discussed in this book are very helpful in protecting your immune system against infections.

NUTRITIONAL SUPPORT. Although mentioned last, this is the most important part of treatment, because it supports your body in healing itself. This is why the book you are holding focuses on healing your body nutritionally!

Foods That Fight Fibromyalgia will empower you to begin your healing process. It will also give you a number of tools to improve your diet. I would add one caveat, however: Everyone is different, and although we can tell you which foods are most likely to help, individual needs vary considerably. Therefore, in applying Deirdre's suggestions and guidelines (or anyone else's, including mine), tune in to your body, to see how they make you feel. Continue to apply those that leave you feeling better, and feel free to discontinue the others.

Discouraged and worried that you simply cannot get well? Let's look at the data, so you can discard that misconception. Our study, entitled "Effective Treatment of CFS and Fibromyalgia" (*Journal of CFS*, see full text at www.endfatigue.com), in which we used SHIN, showed that 91 percent of patients improved with treatment, with an average improvement in quality of life of 90 percent. Many patients no longer even qualified for a diagnosis of fibromyalgia or CFS following treatment. In support of our work, an editorial in the *Journal of the American Academy of Pain Management* (the largest multidisciplinary society of pain specialists in the United States) noted: "The comprehensive and aggressive metabolic approach to treatment detailed in the Teitelbaum study are all highly successful approaches and make fibromyalgia a very treatment-responsive disorder. The study by Dr. Teitelbaum et al. and years of clinical experience

make this approach an excellent and powerfully effective part of the standard of practice for treatment of people who suffer from fibromyalgia and myofascial pain syndrome."

Although this book focuses primarily on diet, it also provides other pertinent information for healing. For example, Chapter 12 discusses other helpful nutrients that are powerful tools for improving health. Our recently published study shows that use of a nutrient called D-ribose (the study used Corvalen by Bioenergy) is a major step forward in treating fatigue in the average fibromyalgia/CFS patient, resulting in a 44.7 percent improvement in energy after two to three weeks. In our study, pain, sleep difficulty, and "brain fog" also improved.

At this time, research has proven that you have all the tools you need to get well. This book will help you do this! I wish you all of God's blessings and best wishes in your healing.

—Jacob Teitelbaum, M.D.

Dr. Teitelbaum is a board-certified internist and medical director of the national chain of Fibromyalgia and Fatigue Centers. Having suffered with and overcome these illnesses in 1975, he spent the next thirty years creating, researching, and teaching effective therapies for fatigue and pain. He is the senior author of the landmark studies "Effective Treatment of Chronic Fatigue Syndrome and Fibromyalgia— a Placebo-Controlled Study" and "Effective Treatment of CFS and Fibromyalgia with D-Ribose." Dr. Teitelbaum lectures internationally and is the author of the best-selling book From Fatigued to Fantastic!: A Clinically Proven Program to Regain Vibrant Health and Overcome Chronic Fatigue and Fibromyalgia *and* Pain Free 1-2-3: A Proven Program for Eliminating Chronic Pain *Now. His website can be found at www.endfatigue.com.*

INTRODUCTION

If you are reading this book, you are probably already in the battle against fibromyalgia and chronic pain, or you may be supporting someone who is. You may also have been living with this battle for some time, coping with a variety of crippling physical and emotional symptoms for which you have not yet found relief. Or perhaps you are part of someone else's struggle, a close family member or friend with fibromyalgia, and you are helping them find answers. In any event, you are looking for ways to heal and become well again—goals that are possible and within your reach.

If you have fibromyalgia, you are fully aware of the havoc it can wreak on your health and well-being—the array of debilitating symptoms, from pain and fatigue to depression and insomnia. Although fibromyalgia is not life-threatening, making the basic decisions and choices that are a part of everyday life can be consumed by the need to survive mentally, physically, and emotionally from day to day. Ordinary life becomes a battlefield, and even simple things are no longer simple. Instead, chronic pain and fatigue are behind every thought and action, and relief, when it arrives, is often short-lived and transient. Moving from a place in which living with pain is a typical part of your day to one that is pain-free and energized is a goal worth pursuing, and it is within your grasp. You can take heart from knowing that *Foods That Fight Fibromyalgia* provides you with sound knowledge and practical tools to aid you in your recovery process.

Eating the right foods is essential to your recovery from fibromyalgia—and to your overall health and longevity. *Foods That Fight Fibromyalgia* gives you powerful nutritional tools to help secure a healthy future.

Part I offers basic food and nutrition guidelines to lead you toward health and healing—for example, emphasis on eating whole foods and avoiding "anti-nutrients," such as highly processed or pesticide and chemically laden options. Obtaining a balanced level of healthy proteins, carbohydrates, and fats at each meal is not only important for maintaining energy but is also essential for healthy hormones and metabolism and to stabilize weight. Moreover, it is important to supply the body with several essential daily nutrients in which many people

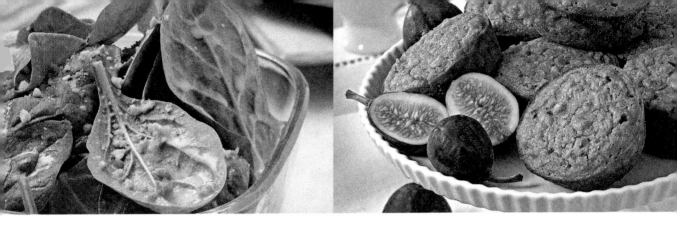

with fibromyalgia are deficient. These, plus the nutritional supplements you can take to obtain these nutrients, will be discussed in detail.

In Part II of this book, you will find a wealth of recipes that have been specially selected and designed to help you in your recovery from fibromyalgia. In addition to helping you heal and recover, continued use of the recipes can provide ongoing support to your health and well-being. You will have learned new and healthier eating habits to aid in your continued success.

To ensure that you always choose the best foods for every meal or snack, and to provide you with optimal ways of knowing how to make healthy selections, each recipe is followed by a "Health Facilitator" rating. This rating chart enables you to plan meals and snacks that are well-balanced and contain sufficiently high levels of all the important nutrients and components necessary to healthy eating. Each recipe has been rated according to its balance level and its protein, fat, and carbohydrate, as well as fiber, antioxidant, and enzyme, content.

Foods That Fight Fibromyalgia includes the most up-to-date nutritional information currently available. After reading and following the principles in this book, you will understand some of the basics of the body's biochemistry and the necessity for revising your personal nutrition. This will bring about positive change that extends beyond your immediate condition to provide you with maximum health benefits.

The payoff from implementing a personally focused healthy eating program extends far beyond warding off symptoms. It can also bring about a significant improvement in every area of your health and the quality of life that good health affords.

Rest assured that your recovery from fibromyalgia is an attainable goal and that this book is designed with that goal clearly in mind. I wish you enhanced vitality, long life, and good health while you continue your journey of recovery and move towards high-level wellness.

PART I

UNDERSTANDING FIBROMYALGIA

CHAPTER 1

THE CAUSES AND THE CURES

Fibromyalgia is a collection of symptoms that include pain, stiffness, and tenderness of the muscles, tendons, joints, and other soft tissues. As a chronic condition, it results in a system that is exhausted and overloaded. In fibromyalgia, there is a generalized disturbance in pain processing that produces "pain amplification"—that is, fibromyalgia patients experience pain in response to stimuli that would not ordinarily be painful for healthy people. In addition to pain and tenderness, fibromyalgia is characterized by fatigue, restless sleep, feeling tired upon awakening, morning stiffness, headaches, dizziness, trouble concentrating, depression, anxiety, and inactivity. It has been associated with stress, tension, trauma, overexertion, hormone deficiency diseases (particularly thyroid disease), alterations in brain chemistry (which can result from malnutrition and poor dietary habits), anemia, parasites, and viral infections.

Fibromyalgia is technically a syndrome and not a disease, since by definition diseases tend to have known causes and well-understood mechanisms that produce symptoms. The term *syndrome* refers to an association of several clinically recognizable features, signs, symptoms, or characteristics that occur together. While fibromyalgia has a recurring set of symptoms, its exact cause is not completely known yet, and it is therefore categorized as a syndrome.

What Causes Fibromyalgia?

Although there has been considerable international investigation devoted to understanding fibromyalgia, no single cause factor has yet been identified. Because experts in the field disagree on its causes, fibromyalgia is often classified as a rheumatic disorder, similar in origin to rheumatoid arthritis, or it is described as an autoimmune disorder because it often develops along with other conditions, such as chronic fatigue syndrome (CFS) or lupus erythematosus. Unlike the stiffness of rheumatoid arthritis, the pain from fibromyalgia typically doesn't diminish with activity, and the pain is made worse by cold, damp weather, overexertion, anxiety, or stress.

It is also firmly established that a central nervous system dysfunction is primarily responsible for the increased pain sensitivity that often comes with fibromyalgia. Dysfunction in the nervous system can lead to thyroid and adrenal problems and other hormonal abnormalities, which are common findings in many people with fibromyalgia. In any event, fibromyalgia leaves the sufferer with a wide range of symptom fluctuations and high levels of debilitating pain, which can be so disabling that at least 30 percent of sufferers cannot sustain customary lifestyles and occupations due to the unrelenting exhaustion and depletion of their energy and vitality.

Researchers studying fibromyalgia patients have found irregularities in their spinal fluid and a relatively low level of the brain chemical serotonin. In the central nervous system, serotonin is believed to play an important role in the regulation of our moods, sleep, impulses, appetites, and motivations. Low levels of serotonin are associated with several other disorders in addition to fibromyalgia, including clinical depression, bipolar disorder, anxiety disorders, and irritable bowel syndrome. The food you eat has the potential to raise or lower your serotonin levels. That's why the ingredients in a particular meal have a powerful impact on the way you feel after you eat.

The body makes serotonin out of an amino acid called tryptophan. Amino acids are the building blocks of protein, and tryptophan is found in abundance in all high-protein foods, such as dairy products, eggs, meat, and fish. Vegetarian foods, including seeds, nuts, and a number of vegetables, also offer many good sources of tryptophan. When these foods are digested, their amino acids, including tryptophan, enter the bloodstream and are carried to tissues that use them to synthesize the body's own proteins and other essential molecules, including serotonin. Of all the chemicals present in the brain, serotonin is probably the most important for maintaining a sensation of well-being, which explains why serotonin is known as Mother Nature's "feel-good chemical." Chapter 4 examines serotonin in more detail and suggests

the best food sources for raising serotonin levels and lifting moods.

Fibromyalgia patients suffer from a definite lowering of the immune system defenses, which can leave the door open to invading bacteria, viruses, and infections. Often, we aren't aware that our body is shifting into defense mode to fight off a virus or bacteria that's attacking. Fibromyalgia can be brought on by a combination of triggers, such as stress, toxins, infections, and diet, so it's vital to improve your health on every level to build the immune system back up. You will learn many ways in which to accomplish that in this book.

Who Is Affected by Fibromyalgia?

Fibromyalgia is widespread, affecting between 6 and 15 percent of the adult population in the United States, and it is most commonly diagnosed in individuals between the ages of twenty and fifty. It may occur at any age, though, even in childhood, and is seven times more common in women than in men. The current incidence of fibromyalgia in women is approximately 3.5 percent and increases with age to more than 7 percent between the ages of 60 and 79.

Common Medical Treatments for Fibromyalgia

Although the American Medical Association (AMA) recognized fibromyalgia as an illness and a major cause of disability in 1987, many physicians today still lack the skills to diagnose and treat it effectively. Diagnosis is difficult because the symptoms are so diverse and vary among sufferers. This can delay the onset of treatment and curative measures and drive the patient into a downward spiral of despair and depression. For most, a timely and accurate diagnosis of the problem offers tremendous relief. It helps to finally learn what the condition is, to know that it's a recognized illness, and to get confirmation that it's not "just in your head."

Physicians usually offer fibromyalgia patients a variety of pharmaceutical drugs, including pain relievers, non-steroidal anti-inflammatory drugs (NSAIDs), muscle relaxants, tranquilizers, serotonin re-uptake inhibitors (SRIs), and antidepressants. While they may offer temporary relief of some symptoms, none has had any long-term benefits or proven particularly helpful in the majority of cases. Attempts to focus on a specific set of symptoms, such as aches and stiffness, for example, are counterproductive because these are symptoms of an insidious life problem that must be solved at its source. To date, no one has been cured of fibromyalgia through drugs alone. Medicine and drugs are most effective when they are combined with a change in diet and the addition of proper nutritional support, patient education, stress reduction, lifestyle modification techniques, and regular exercise. Research studies have verified that the best outcomes result from a combination of approaches that address the problem at its source and that diet and nutrition are major factors in sourcing and solving the problem.

Associated Disorders

A number of other disorders produce many of the same symptoms as fibromyalgia. These include the following:

- Chronic fatigue syndrome
- Irritable bowel syndrome
- Lupus erythematosus
- Myofascial pain syndrome
- Tension myositis syndrome
- Mercury toxicity
- Lyme disease
- Influenza
- Gulf War syndrome
- Thyroid disease
- Tendonitis
- Vitamin B12 deficiency
- Vitamin D deficiency
- Lead poisoning
- Depression

- Carpal tunnel syndrome
- Mitral valve prolapse
- Raynaud's syndrome
- Rheumatic disease

It is unusual to see a fibromyalgia sufferer who does not exhibit another health problem. Greater than 60 percent of patients diagnosed with fibromyalgia have chronic digestive disorders, and more than half have symptoms suggestive of allergies to food and airborne allergens. Many are overweight and have blood sugar abnormalities. They present with an obvious biochemical upset and imbalance, which leads us again to nutrition and the need for closely scrutinizing our diet.

Energy Loss

Fibromyalgia is akin to an energy crisis: One of the major complaints expressed by people diagnosed with the disorder is a feeling of complete and utter exhaustion and total lack of energy and vitality. In support of this theory, studies have found that fibromyalgia patients suffer from a condition in which structures called mitochondria within the muscle cells are inefficient in their production of energy, causing fatigue and a loss of energy and vitality. The lack of cellular energy eventually leads to immune system dysfunction. This is because the immune system is missing the energy it needs to eliminate toxins from the body or to fight infections. The immune system, already in a weakened state, is put under even more stress, leading to further exhaustion.

Nutrient deficiencies are another common finding in people who have problems maintaining or sustaining energy levels or who complain of feeling chronically tired. Our body requires a minimum of at least fifty vitamins and minerals every day. To get them, we need not only to eat a properly balanced diet but also to take vitamin and mineral supplements to replenish these stores and build up reserves. All people with fibromyalgia have some form of nutrient deficiency combined with decreased absorption capabilities. Gastrointestinal tract problems are especially common. They typically result from dysbiosis (better known as leaky gut syndrome, which is explained in Chapter 3) or enzyme deficiencies from eating too many processed foods, chemical sensitivity, hormonal imbalances, and stress. These underlying gastrointestinal tract problems make it all the more important to examine the nutritional habits and practices of anyone suffering from fibromyalgia.

It is not surprising that nutrition plays a significant role in supplying energy to cells, when you consider that a common denominator of low energy is faulty blood sugar metabolism—sometimes called reactive or functional hypoglycemia. Hypoglycemia (also known as low blood sugar), occurs when your blood glucose (blood sugar) level drops too low to provide enough energy for your body's activities. Symptoms result from sugar levels fluctuating and swinging from high to low. This leaves you feeling fatigued and you may develop food cravings, particularly for sweets, alcohol, or caffeinated drinks. Mood swings, drowsiness, mental confusion, depression, and impaired memory and concentration are just a few of the mental symptoms that can result, because your brain is literally being starved of glucose, which it needs for fuel. When consumed in excess, sugar and high-glycemic carbohydrates can wreak havoc on your body and, in particular, your immune system. It can lead to insulin resistance and eventually to diabetes (the fifth leading cause of death in the United States).

Moreover, the source of the problem—be it hypoglycemia or fibromyalgia—is strongly influenced by improper diet and poor nutrition. Nutritional deficiencies and bad habits, such as smoking, eating too many refined and processed foods, and excessive caffeine and alcohol consumption, can contribute to the onset of fibromyalgia. The good news is that proper nutrition and improved lifestyle habits can also help you overcome it! There

is comfort in knowing that the body has a near-miraculous capacity to heal and recover.

In later chapters, we will discuss in more detail the most vital nutrients, vitamins, and minerals that can help you win the battle against fibromyalgia and regain optimum health.

Summary

- No single cause factor has yet been identified for fibromyalgia, and many sufferers exhibit other disorders.
- It has been firmly established that a central nervous system dysfunction is responsible for the increased pain sensitivity that often accompanies fibromyalgia.
- Fibromyalgia occurs at any age, even in childhood, and is seven times more common in women than in men.
- All people with fibromyalgia have some form of nutrient deficiency.
- Serotonin, a "feel-good" chemical, is relatively low in people with fibromyalgia, affecting mood, sleep, impulses, appetites, and motivations. The body makes serotonin from an amino acid called tryptophan. Tryptophan is found in foods such as turkey, eggs, dairy, seeds, nuts, and a number of fruits and vegetables.
- Nutrition plays a large role in supplying energy to cells.
- More than 60 percent of patients diagnosed with fibromyalgia have chronic digestive disorders and food allergies.
- It is essential to include nutritional strategies in your battle plan against fibromyalgia.
- Fibromyalgia can be reversed by making appropriate nutrition and healthy lifestyle choices.

CHAPTER 2

FIGHTING FIBROMYALGIA THROUGH DIET

Like most chronic conditions, fibromyalgia develops gradually over time—usually several years. Upon close inspection, the health background and history of sufferers often reveal a number of long-term, chronic, or recurrent symptoms that have built up and appeared over time. They may have been symptoms that were earlier dismissed or discounted. We tend not to link symptoms together or to see them as potential elements in a complex dysfunctional, and generally declining, state of health. As symptoms stabilize, we go about our lives with diminished function or slowly increasing disability. Add to the mix any stress factors, such as the birth of a new baby, moving to a new home, taking a new job, or having an accident that requires hospitalization and drug therapy, and suddenly our bodies can no longer cope.

For many people, increased levels of stress translate into coping behaviors and strategies that actually make matters worse. For example, they may respond by drinking more coffee and/or alcohol, eating junk foods, smoking cigarettes, working longer hours, and exercising less or not at all. They might reassure themselves that everything "is okay in an effort to deny that their health is steadily declining. Highly motivated, goal-oriented, type-A personalities are likely to respond in this

manner, and in our fast-paced world, many people's lives are supercharged and filled with more than enough to handle on a daily basis. They stretch, over a period of time, beyond a manageable range, until finally they are diagnosed with a disabling condition or chronic disease. It is not a sudden onset of illness in an otherwise perfectly healthy body but rather the end result of a downward-spiraling series of negative events and symptoms occurring over months or even years. After a lengthy period of sending obvious signs of distress, the body finally collapses under all the pressure.

Even if you accept that there is no distinct starting point for fibromyalgia but rather that it gradually creeps up over time, you may still be asking what brought it on.

Many patients with fibromyalgia report pain-precipitating events, particularly physical or emotional traumas, infections, or surgeries. These stressors often act as triggers that result in high degrees of pain, life interference, decreased levels of physical activity, and even complete disability.

Although cases exist of Fibromyalgia in children, whose parents—one or both—suffer from fibromyalgia, the condition is not classified solely as hereditary. It may be tempting to make genetics the main culprit and blame your personal luck of the draw in the genetic lottery, but this would not be a fitting explanation. The majority of people with fibromyalgia do not come from families with the disorder. How your genes express themselves depends on factors within your control—in particular, diet and lifestyle.

Genes and Your Health

Many people believe that genes have a big hand in determining their fate and that they are stuck with what they inherited from their parents. In other words, if your mother had breast cancer, your grandfather got Alzheimer's in his 60s, or your father has diabetes, then, chances are, you will, too, and there's nothing much you can do about it. The truth is that, while our genes may predispose us toward certain illnesses, we are not necessarily fated to have them. We can change the way our genes are expressed, and we do this already through our daily choices in lifestyle habits and nutrition.

Scientists have now confirmed that even though a gene for a specific tendency or disease may exist, its expression is subject to environmental factors—both external and nutritional. This means that we can influence which genes get turned on or off by changing our environment. What we eat by way of essential nutrients in our diet influences gene expression. This means that your individual genetic variation and expression of your genes is dependent upon your diet and lifestyle. The problem, however, is that we tend to inherit our parents' lifestyles and their habits along with their genes. This includes the foods we eat and those we don't, and it often leads to the same conditions and health challenges that they faced.

Genetic predisposition toward fibromyalgia—or any disease condition—is mainly determined by the environment in which your genes function. Your genes express themselves based on nutrients (macronutrients, micronutrients, air, water) and lifestyle factors, of which diet plays a central role.

In the cell, gene expression results in the manufacture of proteins that determine an organism's characteristics, including its health and ability to function optimally, as well as its survival rate. The study of the interaction between nutrition and genes is a highly innovative and fast-growing field.

Two new sciences explore this territory: nutritional genomics (or nutrigenomics) and epigenetics. Nutrigenomics combines information from genetics, nutrition, physiology, pathology, molecular biology, and other scientific disciplines and links the response to changes in type and concentration of dietary chemicals and the understanding of their effects on health.

It is now accepted that nutrients alter molecular processes, such as DNA structure, gene expression, and metabolism, and that these processes in turn may initiate disease and contribute to its progression. Individual genetic variation can influence how nutrients are assimilated, metabolized, stored, and excreted by the body.

Epigenetics explores the relationship between proteins and genes and studies how genes can be turned on and off by chemical reactions from changes in the proteins that bond to the DNA. These proteins can be altered by environmental factors such as heavy chemicals or nutrition.

Although this science is being used in connection to cancer treatment, it provides us with a clear understanding of how our genetic blueprint is affected by our environment and nutritional intake—which comes as welcome news because nutrition is something we can do something about!

The Link Between Diet, Nutrition, and Fibromyalgia

It's common knowledge now that diet is an important factor in the onset and proliferation of human disease, as well as in its prevention. Chemicals in food interact with biochemical pathways at the molecular level and demonstrate a direct cause-and-effect relationship between health and disease. For example, the use of fumigants, pesticides, and insecticides for growing fruits and vegetables can damage the nervous system, respiratory system, kidneys, liver, and heart. Synthetics used in the production of meats, such as antibiotics, hormones, and tranquilizers, challenge the immune system and contribute to hormone imbalances in humans. Antibiotics can also reduce the friendly flora in the digestive tract. Research has shown that certain strains of bacteria have built up resistance to antibiotics, allowing unfriendly organisms to thrive unchecked.

Increasing evidence points to diet and nutrition as major players in the reduction of fibromyalgia symptoms. Some of the latest fibromyalgia and other rheumatic or immune compromised disorder therapies rely on nutrition and diet modification. In fact, including or excluding specific foods is one of the most successful approaches used today.

The role of diet and nutrition in treating fibromyalgia has been the subject of a small but growing body of research, with results showing benefits in pain reduction, sleep quality, and general health. Removing anti-nutrients from the diet (caffeine, alcohol, sugar, preservatives, chemicals, and others) and adding foods high in antioxidants, minerals, and vitamins derived from a raw or live-foods vegetarian/vegan diet have produced a marked increase in quality of health in every case.

By improving the diet with balanced nutrition, we help address fibromyalgia at its source and prevent burdening the body with chemicals or toxic elements that may weaken it further. Even mainstream medicine agrees. According to the National Institutes of Health, "Foods contain nutrients essential for normal metabolic function, and when problems arise, they result from imbalances in nutrient intake and from harmful interaction with other factors." In addition to being poten-

tially effective, implementing proper nutrition and dietary modifications is an easy and comparatively low-cost treatment method.

Dangers of the American Lifestyle

We are witnessing an unprecedented epidemic of chronic degenerative diseases in the United States—one that is directly related to the foods we eat and the way we live. Every fourth person in North America is the victim of one or more degenerative conditions. Almost half the population of the United States and Canada are subject to a variety of physical or mental illnesses. These recurrently sick people fall prey to chronic diseases that range from learning and behavioral disorders in children and age-related diseases such as arthritis and Alzheimer's, to general feelings of lethargy and drained energy. There is hope, however, and it can be found in your diet.

The explosive rise in the incidence of chronic degenerative disease exists, despite an enormous expenditure of resources and the stunning technological advances made over the past sixty years. Fibromyalgia and chronic fatigue syndrome are two of the fastest growing degenerative diseases present in every developing country that has adopted the Western lifestyle. Worldwide, more than 29 million deaths a year are caused by these chronic lifestyle diseases. In 2000, the number of people with chronic health conditions was 20 million more than the number projected in 1996. In America today, there are more than 125 million people with chronic illness—a number that is expected to reach 157 million people by 2020.

Coping with a complex chronic illness such as fibromyalgia affects both individuals and their families. Life for these people can seem like a relentless struggle against disabling conditions that lead eventually to immobility, senility, or death. There is a demonstrable link between advances in technology, primarily in the agro-business sector, and deteriorating health and wellness in our society. There is also a direct correlation between the drive for corporate profits and the rampant obesity now prevalent in Western society.

Americans' gradually deteriorating health is due, in part, to the consumption of artificial foods lacking in natural vitamins and minerals. Processed food manufacturers have dissipated and distorted nature's quality control by removing nutrients and adding artificial substances and flavorings—most notably, and most detrimentally, sugar. Almost twenty years ago, the Surgeon General's Report on Health and Nutrition ranked "what we eat" as the "one personal choice which seems to influence long-term health prospects more than any other, for adult Americans who do not smoke and do not drink excessively."

Many people with chronic diseases continue to eat poorly, failing to realize that their food choices are contributing to their ill health. Nutritional counseling is a topic that is seldom discussed by many medical practitioners— although a wave of acceptance of the benefits of proper nutrition has begun in Europe, particularly in Germany, where upward of 80 percent of doctors regularly prescribe herbs, vitamins, and other supplements to their patients as a necessary starting point and move on to drugs only as a last resort.

Fibromyalgia and chronic fatigue syndrome are products of the new American diet and way of life. If we are to succeed at overcoming them, it's up to us to take deliberate steps to reverse the conditions and environments that caused them. And the first steps involve our diet and nutrition. We need food that nourishes, that tastes good, and that we can savor and enjoy while it works with, rather than against, our biology and our genes.

It's True: You Are What You Eat

Research continues to confirm the adage that we are what we eat. Consequently, where health is a concern, then the food we eat is the ultimate medicine. What we eat provides the fuel our body uses to build cells, tissues, and organs. The atoms in a carrot, for example, will take their place in the new cells being built. The carrot's atoms may become part of skin cells, muscle cells, or blood cells. In addition to using food to build cells and tissues, food provides the energy an organism needs to stay alive. Food provides our matter (what we are made of) and our energy (what keeps us alive). So we really are what we eat.

The scientific community is virtually unanimous in its belief that changes in diet and improved nutrition can increase a person's health and help prevent chronic diseases and degenerative conditions. In fact, there is no drug, vitamin pill, herb, or other nutritional supplement that can influence your health as profoundly as your diet. It is estimated that at least seven of the top ten causes of death can be positively affected by an improved diet.

Despite the compelling evidence, however, we have great difficulty adhering to what makes sense. We consume the elements of our own destruction and dig our graves with knives and forks. We do this through an excessive intake of sugar, hydrogenated fats and oils, and processed foods that lack fiber and are devoid of any nutritional content. We fall victim to television-advertising or headlines proclaiming that certain foods offer health benefits or that certain other foods threaten ill effects, causing us to react—at least in the short term. We give up red meat, fill up on fiber, and start popping pills containing the synthetic version of the latest "health" food in an attempt to apply a quick-fix solution before resuming our usual daily habits and lifestyles. These impulsive reactions are like searching for a magic potion, and they yield results that are equally disappointing.

The answer, therefore, is not in a short-run, quick-fix, single-focus deprivation diet, nor is it in a magic potion or pill. There is simply no alternative to a fundamental and lasting change in diet that will bring about improved health. The good news is that making the change to a healthful diet is not difficult. For at the center of this new way of eating are foods that contain all the necessary nutrients filled with vitamins, minerals, fiber, and enzymes to ensure optimal health. These foods are drawn chiefly from fruits, vegetables, grains, legumes, nuts, and seeds that are readily accessible and versatile enough to yield an almost limitless number of dishes. The evidence continues to mount that these foods deliver what just may be—if anything can be—elixirs of long life and good health.

Increasing Cellular Energy

Studies show that poor cellular energy production due to poisoning of the energy-producing machinery of the cell (the mitochondria) is a characteristic common to both fibromyalgia and chronic fatigue syndrome. In studies at the Abington Memorial Hospital in Pennsylvania, rheumatology researchers found that fibromyalgia patients suffered from a condition loosely described as "muscle toxicity," in which the mitochondria within muscle cells were inefficiently producing energy. In addition, people with fibromyalgia were seen to have smaller than normal muscle fibers that exhibited misshapen mitochondria not found in normal subjects.

A Swedish study showed that poor energy status of muscles in fibromyalgia may be due to reduced blood flow to the affected tissue, which can lead directly to reduced tissue oxygenation, lower energy reserves, and poor oxidative capacity. Reduced energy is generally associated with a decrease in the total concentration of energy in the cell, meaning there is simply not enough energy to fuel the full range of cellular functions. The additional complication of poor mitochondrial function and diminished glucose metabolism, which both lower energy reserves, suggests that muscles in people with fibromyalgia are energy-starved.

Mitochondria are the same parts of the cell that are involved in producing energy during exercise. When excess exercise causes fatigue, and you develop muscle pain, you have exceeded the ability of your cells' mitochondria to generate energy effectively. Waste products accumulate in the mitochondria, poisoning their function. At this point, fatigue rapidly sets in. Chronic fatigue and people with fibromyalgia experience feelings of extreme fatigue, as if they had done strenuous exercise—but without any exertion. Increasing cellular energy through nutrition can help relax tense muscles and interrupt the downward spiral of overwhelming fatigue, soreness, and stiffness.

Unraveling the mystery of fibromyalgia uncovers a complex interplay of causative factors that contribute to the condition and the low energy and devastating fatigue that take hold. According to interviews with hundreds of patients with fibromyalgia and chronic fatigue syndrome, nearly all are nutritionally depleted and have immune dysfunction. Common denominators among fibromyalgia patients are:

- Extreme fatigue and low energy
- Metabolism abnormalities
- Food allergies
- Digestive dysfunction and poor absorption
- Exposure to toxins (such as mercury, cadmium, aluminum, and lead)
- Chronic infections that could be fungal, bacterial, viral, or even parasitic
- Immune system dysfunction

Fatigue

Fatigue is a symptom associated with many ailments and is among the first signals our body sends urging us to pay attention to our health. We can respond by providing the body with adequate rest, not smoking, avoiding toxins and chemicals that pollute us, exercising and deep breathing, drinking plenty of clean water, and giving the body all the nutrients it needs to convert food into energy. Our goal in the pursuit of health and higher energy levels is to understand where our energy comes from and to practice habits that restore and strengthen rather than weaken the body.

Many people respond to a decline in energy by using stimulants, such as coffee, sugar, alcohol, cigarettes, and over-the-counter or illicit drugs. These only worsen the problem by burdening the liver's detoxification ability. They can also lead to a host of other, more serious, system breakdowns and health-related problems. To achieve consistent levels of energy, you must rid the body of toxins, while increasing nutrients to optimal levels. It stands to reason that we accumulate energy by building the body up and not by destroying it further.

One of the first questions to ask in your quest for more energy and less fatigue is what is slowing you down. Many things get in the way of energy production, including:

- A build-up of toxins throughout the body
- A diet lacking in proper nutrients
- High levels of stress; adrenal exhaustion
- Prescription and over-the-counter medications
- Food allergies and sensitivities
- Impaired liver function
- Deficiencies in vitamins, minerals, and essential fatty acids
- Overgrowth of yeast or fungus in the GI tract
- Impaired thyroid function
- Trauma (including physical, mental, and emotional)
- Parasites
- Insufficient exercise
- Not enough sleep

When our cells and immune system are under attack, a great deal of our available energy reserves are used to boost immune function. In a healthy body, the average person consumes enough nutrition daily to sustain health. In a less than healthy body or one that's under attack, we need more than our normal daily requirements to stay healthy—we need additional nutrients to protect our cells and compounds that specifically target pathogens. In the following chapters, we will discuss energy-enhancing nutrients and supplements, particularly those designed to combat fatigue conditions like fibromyalgia. By neutralizing free radicals that interfere with metabolism, as well as those given off by the body as part of everyday metabolism, ingesting the right nutrients makes all the difference. And staying clear of anti-nutrients and environmental toxins that deplete and drain us of energy, particularly when our body's health is already compromised, is essential.

Decreasing Anti-Nutrients— the Energy Drainers

Anti-nutrients are substances that directly interfere with the absorption of vitamins, minerals, and other nutrients. To some degree, we are all exposed to them through our food and water supplies. For example, some plant-derived food ingredients—such as enzyme inhibitors, saponins, lectins, and phytic acid—have been identified as anti-nutrients. At high concentrations, some are toxic, but at lower levels, some of these plant-derived compounds can be beneficial. However, the anti-nutrients referred to in this discussion are those that antagonize the nutrients we need for good health. Sugar, food coloring, trans fats, additives like BHT, and most of the more than 3,500 food additives and preservatives allowed in the United States should be viewed as anti-nutrients.

Some anti-nutrients bind to other nutrients, rendering them useless. Others tie up enzymes needed in digestion and other body functions. Drugs and pharmaceutical medications cause problems by depleting nutrients and thereby creating an even greater need for certain essential nutrients. Other anti-nutrients cause nutrients to be excreted more rapidly from the body. Cell phones, electromagnetic fields, modern technology, and high stress levels can all contribute to the level of anti-nutrients to which we are exposed.

Many of the anti-nutrients damage your cells' mitochondria, robbing your body of vital energy and leaving you fatigued and lethargic. They also have a direct or indirect effect on immune function and compromise your body's ability to repel infections and other potential invaders. Many of today's diseases are caused as much by an excess of anti-nutrients as by a deficiency of nutrients. Health problems such as fibromyalgia and chronic fatigue syndrome can follow from an influx of anti-nutrients that exceeds the body's capacity to detoxify. Once this threshold is exceeded, toxins such as pesticide residues accumulate in fat tissue, common drugs from painkillers to alcohol become increasingly toxic, and we eventually experience muscle aches, pain, and extreme fatigue.

Most junk foods can be classified as anti-nutrients, because the body requires more nutrients to process and to make use of them than the junk food provides. Whatever you can do to reduce your exposure to anti-nutrients and increase your levels of nutrients will help prevent recurring illness and restore optimum health. We will suggest the ways in which you can accomplish this in the following chapters.

Pesticides and Immune System Dysfunction

Many pesticides and chemicals are so widespread that we are unaware of them. But they have worked their way into our bodies faster than they can be eliminated, and they are causing allergies, chronic fatigue, immune system dysfunction and deficiencies, and energy depletion at record levels. Certain chemicals interact with human DNA, so long-term exposure may result in metabolic and genetic alteration that affects cell growth and behavior.

The U.S. Environmental Protection Agency (EPA) defines a pesticide as "any substance or mixture of substances intended for preventing, destroying, repelling, or mitigating any pest." This includes substances that kill weeds (herbicides), insects (insecticides), fungus (fungicides), rodents (rodenticides), and others. Pesticides can be found in the air we breathe, the food we eat, and the water we drink. They can be a chemical or they may be biologically based. Many pesticides are poisonous to humans and other mammals. In the words of the EPA, "Pesticides are not 'safe.' They are produced specifically because they are toxic to something."

Pesticide exposure is associated with depression, trouble with memory, mood destabilization, and aggressive outbursts. Research by the World Health Organization and the National Cancer Institute implicates environmental chemicals in at least 60 to 80 percent of all cancers. These findings mean that most cancers could be prevented by minimizing or eliminating our exposure to chemicals carcinogens.

It's a well-established fact that our immune systems are under stress from our modern-day, high-tech, chemically-dependent lifestyles. Fibromyalgia is one of the health consequences of a weakened immune system. Others include increased frequency and duration of colds and flu; allergies; asthma; autoimmune disorders such as arthritis, lupus, and diabetes; and chronic fatigue syndrome. It is therefore critical to identify and remove from our environment all sources of toxic substances that have the potential to suppress immune function.

Water—Quality and Quantity

Water is an essential part of a healthy diet. Approximately 60 to 70 percent of our body is composed of water, and it is involved in virtually every bodily function, including circulation, digestion, the assimilation and absorption of nutrients, and the elimination of body wastes. Water is also the main transporter of nutrients throughout the body, via fluids such as blood, lymph, urine, tears, digestive juices, and sweat. Water carries electrolytes, such as sodium, calcium, magnesium, and potassium, which are needed to convey electrical currents in the body. Because water is continually being eliminated through urine and sweating, we must replenish our supply by drinking water throughout the day.

Drinking quality water is necessary to recover from every disorder known to mankind. Water helps flush toxins from the body, and if not enough water is consumed, they can build up in the system, causing a variety of symptoms, such as headaches, nausea, vomiting, and diarrhea. Disorders such as chronic fatigue syndrome and fibromyalgia require plenty of clean water daily, to help flush out toxins and other substances that accumulate in the body and contribute to muscle aches and extreme fatigue. Insufficient water consumption can contribute to various health problems, such as joint and muscle soreness, poor muscle tone, digestive problems, and poor functioning of many organs. Consuming plenty of water can slow the aging process and prevent or alleviate arthritis, kidney stones, constipation, hypoglycemia, obesity, and many other diseases. As we age, our sense of thirst becomes dulled, so it is important to drink water throughout the day, even if we don't feel thirsty.

We lose water as a result of metabolism and digestion, as well as through breathing—approximately one pint of liquid is lost each day through exhaling. Drinking coffee, tea, alcohol, and processed beverages doesn't count as hydration for the body. These substances are considered diuretics, meaning they remove more water than they supply, leading to further dehydration. In addition, these substances act as stimulants and add to the toxic load the body is already burdened with when chronic disease exists. It is vital that we drink plenty of quality water—at least eight to ten glasses over the course of a day.

Water has been called the "universal solvent," because it dissolves more substances than any other liquid on Earth. Water's atomic structure—one oxygen atom and two hydrogen atoms—is simple. This structure is also unique in that it produces electrochemical properties, which allow it to create a strong bond with any positively or negatively charged atom. These bonds create density, which allows water to combine with other chemicals to form a solution. Wherever water goes, whether through the ground or through our bodies, it carries with it valuable nutrients, chemicals, sediments, and minerals. Chemical nutrients can then be carried as a solution through runoff into surface water, or infiltrate ground water. Heavy minerals such as salt, calcium, potassium, and zinc can be transported not only through rivers and over land, but through your body, as well.

Other materials carried in suspension or dissolved in water include undesirable contaminants, such as radon, fluoride, arsenic, iron, lead, copper, and other heavy metals that occur naturally. Unnaturally occurring contaminants include fertilizers, asbestos, cyanides, herbicides, pesticides, and industrial chemicals, which can leach into ground water through the soil or into tap water supplies from plumbing pipes. Many of these chemicals have been linked to serious health problems, such as cancer and other chronic conditions. Drinking plenty of fresh pure water from a healthy reliable source cannot be over-emphasized.

For information about local drinking and tap water supplies, the Water Quality Association, which operates a toll-free Safe Drinking Water Hotline, can help you locate an office or laboratory in your area that provides certified water testing. One of the first steps to good nutrition is knowing the origin, processing, and contents of anything we take into our bodies, and water is certainly no exception.

Pharmaceutical Drugs and Nutrient Depletion

People who regularly take medications may not be aware that commonly prescribed drugs can cause nutrient depletion. Scientific studies over the past thirty years have reported on the drug-induced depletion of nutrients. Much of this information, however, has been buried in scientific journals and is only recently coming to light. More than 1,000 commonly prescribed drugs and many over-the-counter medications deplete one or more nutrients in humans, according to the recently published book *The Drug-Induced Nutrient Depletion Handbook.*

This is alarming information, when you consider that millions of Americans regularly eat nutritionally poor diets consisting of junk and processed foods that fail to supply the minimum daily requirement of many essential nutrients. In fact, a nutritional survey sponsored by the U.S. Department of Agriculture reported that 80 percent of Americans do not consume the recommended dietary allowance for one or more of the essential nutrients on a daily basis. Taking drugs when your immune system is already compromised by illness, combined with a nutritionally depleted diet, environmental toxins and pollutants, anti-nutrients, and a high-stress lifestyle only further robs your body of nutrients.

A survey in 1998 revealed that at least twelve of the top twenty medications prescribed in the United States cause nutrient depletions. These include oral contraceptives, anti-ulcer medications, estrogen replacement therapy medications, anti-convulsants, tricyclic antidepressants, antibiotics, beta blockers, phenothiazines, benzodiazepines, and anti-inflammatory, anti-hypertensive, and cholesterol-lowering drugs. Nutrients that are typically depleted through the use of medications, according to *The Drug-Induced Nutrient Depletion Handbook,* include vitamin C, B-complex vitamins, zinc, Co-Q10, vitamin A, vitamin D, calcium, magnesium, potassium, sodium, vitamin K, lactobacillus acidophilus and bifidobacterium, and folic acid.

If you are on medication, make a point to ask your doctor about its effect on your nutrient levels. If your doctor prescribes medication but fails to address its impact on nutrient levels, it may be wise to seek a doctor who will take this into account.

Allergies and Food Chemical Sensitivity

Food allergies and chemical sensitivities are common among people with fibromyalgia. This is easy to accept when, according to James C. Breneman, M.D., former chairman of the Food Allergy Committee of the American College of Allergists, some estimates show more than 60 percent of the population has unknown food intolerances or allergies.

A food allergy is the result of your body's immune system overreacting to food proteins called allergens. Your immune system is the main defense mechanism for fighting infections and deactivating proteins such as food allergens. It does this by identifying foreign invaders and mobilizing the body's white blood cells against them. Some people's immune systems misidentify a nontoxic substance as an invader, and their white blood cells overreact, creating more damage to the body than the nontoxic invader and causing the allergic response to become a disease in itself. Allergic reactions to foods and chemicals typically begin a few minutes to a few hours after eating the offending food, but can sometimes take several days to present.

Food and chemical allergies can trigger a range of symptoms, some of which are behavioral, emotional, and mental. The most common symptoms affect the respiratory system, digestive tract, and skin, and these include sneezing, coughing, wheezing, itching, shortness of breath, nasal congestion, headache, fatigue, hives, and eczema or other skin rashes. They can also cause more severe symptoms, such as panic attacks, compulsive behavior, depression, psychotic episodes, or hallucinations, and they contribute to anxiety, irritability, inability to concentrate, and brain fog. There is a correlation between common symptoms of fibromyalgia, such as fatigue, brain fog, mood swings, insomnia, and headaches, and the fact that they can be caused or worsened by foods. Once the offending food or chemical is identified and eliminated from the diet or environment, a surprisingly large number of people find their allergy symptoms disappear within a short time.

Foods most commonly known to cause allergies include:

- Eggs
- Dairy products, including cow's milk, cheese, butter, yogurt, and ice cream
- Peanuts, Brazil nuts, hazelnuts, and almonds
- Soy beans
- Wheat and gluten, contained in products such as bread, cereal, cookies, and crackers
- Fish and shellfish
- Chocolate
- Coffee, including decaffeinated
- Tea
- Alcohol
- Yeast-based alcohols (beer and wine, but not champagne)
- Citrus fruits
- Corn
- Yeast
- Sugar
- High-fructose corn syrup
- Food additives

The foods most often responsible for non-specific pain or hypersensitivity symptoms in people with fibromyalgia are staple foods such as milk, wheat, eggs, meat, and coffee. You will see some of these ingredients in the recipes that follow in Part II. These foods have been included because they are valuable sources of nutrients—provided, of course, you are not allergic to them.

How to Determine If You Are Allergic

There are three main areas to consider, when determining whether or not your health problems are related to a food allergy or chemical sensitivity: health background and history, symptoms, and allergy testing. If you have a family background or history of allergies, they will more than likely be a significant factor in your present health concerns. If both your parents had or have allergies, your chances of being allergic are approximately 75 percent. If one parent is allergic, or you have relatives on one side of the family with allergies, you have a 30 to 40 percent chance of developing some form of allergy. If neither parent has an apparent allergy, your chances drop to 10 to 15 percent.

If you exhibit one or more of the most common symptoms listed above, it may suggest an allergy or an intolerance to food and chemicals. Additional signs to look for are bags or wrinkles under the eyes, puffy eyes, or patches of dry skin on the face or body.

Several types of diagnostic methods are used in allergy testing, including blood tests, skin tests, pulse testing, muscle testing, and food-elimination tests. Probably the best practical form of testing is a carefully observed and managed elimination diet. This involves eliminating suspected foods from your diet for a period of at least five to ten days before testing begins. Various suspected foods are then reintroduced one at a time, and reactions are noted over the following twenty-four hours. As you add foods back into your diet, keep a diary of any symptoms you experience and monitor your reaction with the pulse test described below.

If, after re-introducing the offending or suspected foods, your symptoms persist, the avoidance period may need to stretch to several weeks or months before trying a small amount of the suspected food. If you have a reaction after a second attempt to reintroduce that particular food into your diet, eliminate it permanently.

The most common signs and symptoms of a true food allergy include: tingling in the mouth; hives, itching or eczema; swelling of the lips, face, tongue and throat, or other parts of the body; wheezing, nasal congestion, or trouble breathing; abdominal pain, diarrhea, nausea, or vomiting; and dizziness, lightheadedness, or fainting. A severe allergic reaction to food—called anaphylaxis— can be life-threatening. Symptoms of anaphylaxis include constriction of airways, including a swollen throat or a lump in your throat that makes it difficult to breathe; shock, with a severe drop in blood pressure; rapid pulse; and loss of consciousness. Emergency treatment is critical in treating anaphylaxis.

Food Rotation

Eating the same foods every day can also lead to the development of food allergies, sensitivities, or intolerances. It's important to also rotate your foods, so that you don't eat the same foods every day. This is crucial, to give your immune system a break and help reverse and prevent a recurrence of a food allergy. Rotating your foods also ensures that you get a full range of vitamins and minerals and helps to avoid boredom and monotony.

Most food allergy tests can identify the foods you need to avoid and those that you can rotate. If your allergy test doesn't specify foods to rotate, you can apply the rotation principle to everything you eat. Avoid eating any of the foods commonly known to cause allergens (see list on page 38) more than once every three to four days for the first three months following the complete exclusion of your allergens. After three months, you can be more flexible, but remain focused on eating a varied diet. Food allergen-free rotation can also lead to dramatic weight loss, often without restriction of calories, because it clears up the allergies that lead to food cravings, overeating, water retention, and a slowed metabolism.

Pulse Testing

Pulse testing can also be an effective and quick way to determine whether or not you are allergic to a certain food. By recording your pulse rate both before and after consuming the food being tested and noting whether your pulse rate increases by at least ten beats per minute, you will know if you are allergic. If you are, omit the offending food from your diet for one month and retest yourself. Muscle testing or kinesiology can also be used to test if a certain food elicits an allergic reaction.

Skin testing and blood testing, provided by your medical practitioner, are more invasive techniques than the do-it-yourself tests described above.

Summary

- Fibromyalgia is brought on by the cumulative effects of our modern lifestyle and diet. The body functions best when we provide it with a proper balance of nutrients and minimize or remove harmful elements. In fact, balance and moderation may be the most important factors in building resistance toward disease and increasing your health and vitality.
- Fibromyalgia does not have a sudden onset. It is the manifestation of a downward spiral effect from a series of negative events and symptoms experienced over months and years.
- The sciences of nutrigenomics and epigenetics explain how our genetic blueprint is modified by our environment and nutritional intake, and they argue for taking control of our long-term health prospects by making sound nutritional choices.

- By improving our diet with balanced nutrition, we address fibromyalgia at its source.
- A gradually deteriorating food supply has been imposed on us by artificial foods deficient in natural vitamins and minerals, modern commercial farming methods, genetic tampering, and the introduction of gross quantities of hormones, antibiotics, and pesticides into the feed-lots and our environment.
- The commercialization of our food supply has introduced heavily processed foods with thousands of artificial preservatives and toxic chemicals, which have made us guinea pigs in a massive uncontrolled experiment, resulting in a declining state of health in North America.
- The evidence is clear: You are what you eat.
- There are no simple answers to what causes fibromyalgia, but we know that nearly all sufferers are nutritionally depleted and have immune dysfunction.
- Anti-nutrients are substances that interfere directly with the absorption of vitamins, minerals, and other nutrients. These can come from household chemicals, pesticides, prescription drugs, and the water supply. They inhibit the body's ability to assimilate nutrition, and they weaken the immune system.
- Food allergies are common amongst people with fibromyalgia and signal the presence of anti-nutrients, which can be as commonplace as the junk foods that fill our diet with artificial sweeteners, high-fructose corn syrup, and hydrogenated oils.

CHAPTER 3

TREATING SYMPTOMS WITH FOOD—NOT PILLS

Medication should never be considered the only form of treatment for fibromyalgia. A holistic strategy is needed—one that incorporates sound nutrition, healthy lifestyle adjustments, and other non-medical strategies for managing the disorder. The term "holistic" refers to a system of health care that emphasizes treatment of the whole person, including analyses of their physical, nutritional, environmental, emotional, social, spiritual, and lifestyle values. Although drugs can offer some short-term symptom relief, they can also cause a host of adverse reactions, which can lead us down a path of increasing health problems and dependence. A holistic approach encompasses all modalities of diagnosis and treatment, including drugs and surgery, if no safer alternatives exist. Holistic medicine focuses on education and personal responsibility for achieving balance and well-being.

For chronic lifestyle illnesses such as fibromyalgia, a magic-bullet drug does not exist, and drugs that are typically prescribed often end up doing more harm than good. The body is an intricate and interconnected network of systems and functions that work on molecular, genetic, and biochemical levels, and it is far more complex than is currently understood by today's scientists and doctors. Therefore,

it's vitally important to take a holistic viewpoint and address the root causes of illness through nutrition to restore balance.

The human body is designed to run on nutrients. It is made up of roughly 65 percent water, 20 percent protein, 13 percent fat, and 2 percent vitamins and minerals. Virtually 100 percent of the body's composition comes from what you eat, drink, and breathe. Every single molecule and cell is built from and fueled by nutrients from the foods you eat and the water you drink. Consequently, eating the highest-quality food in the right quantities is essential for health, vitality, and freedom from disease. When your body develops an acute or chronic illness or disease, it is imperative that you provide it with a complete healing environment, which includes adequate rest, proper nutrition, and removal of the stressors in your life. For your body to heal itself, you need to activate its healing system, which is fully equipped to tackle the problem, rather than relying on medication to counteract the symptoms. Health care resources focus on which medicines to give—rather than on disease prevention or addressing the disease's underlying causes.

For example, when you have high cholesterol and you take a statin drug to lower it, your cholesterol goes down. But when you stop taking the pill, your cholesterol goes right back up. The pill didn't cure the condition; it simply suppressed the high cholesterol. When you take a preventative approach to healing, you seek to eliminate the causes of a particular illness and help the body restore a normal balance, so the illness disappears—for good.

A New Roadmap for Health

Currently, there are no laboratory tests that can confirm a diagnosis of fibromyalgia. For the most part, people with fibromyalgia experience a variety of debilitating symptoms that seem to worsen over time and that often result in an endless series of doctor's visits that bring neither relief nor answers. Fibromyalgia patients cycle through a range of prescriptions and over-the-counter medications, including sleeping pills, antidepressants such as SRIs (serotonin re-uptake inhibitors), NSAIDs (non-steroidal anti-inflammatory drugs), and pain killers. Taking these drugs leads to a cascade of adverse reactions and side effects that weaken health further and can propel the sufferer into depression, deeper exhaustion, and diminishing health.

The simple truth: There is no magic pill. Effective treatment does not consist of a prescription medication or drug. While medication can offer short-term symptom relief, there appears to be a strong link between fibromyalgia and poor diet and nutritional deficiencies. What is critical is changing your lifestyle and living in harmony with your genes. It is a matter of eating foods and nutrients that are nourishing and strengthening, rather than harmful to the body's biochemistry. The body is a biological organism that constantly provides you with feedback. To function and thrive, we must follow some basic rules of biology. These are the laws of nature, and if we don't follow them, we're going to become sick.

At certain times, drugs are necessary and useful, particularly in medical emergencies, but too often drugs are the first choice in treatment, and

they can harm more than heal. Ever more research is revealing that diet, nutrition, environment, lifestyle, habits, attitude, and stress have a profound effect on our immunity and resistance to disease.

If your body is presenting you with symptoms and you've been diagnosed with a chronic disorder, take it as a signal that you need to make very definite changes to your lifestyle. You cannot expect to swallow a magic pill and resume the patterns you had prior to your disorder and get well—that's simply not the way it works. Embrace your diagnosis as an opportunity to make positive changes in your life. You might find the changes difficult to make at first, but, like learning any new habit, they will eventually become natural and fluid. Once they do, though, you will have evolved in a whole new direction that's substantially better—and more healthful—than before.

Connecting Stress to Illness

There is abundant evidence to suggest that fibromyalgia may represent a primary disorder of the autonomic nervous system—meaning that it is stress-related. Many people with fibromyalgia have a history of chronically overdoing it, which can manifest itself in fatigue and muscle pain. These discomforts may reflect emotional and physical stress, which often lead to anxiety and then even more emotional stress. Added emotional stress ratchets up the pain and fatigue, thereby creating more stress, and so the cycle continues.

Stress affects your body as much as does food and exercise. In fact, many people have undetected food allergies that can start the fibromyalgia syndrome ball rolling and place undue stress on the entire body. Prolonged stress weakens us, over time, leaving us susceptible to additional stress, whether physical or emotional. This in turn can trigger a series of downward spiraling health effects, until finally we buckle under all the pressure and become ill. Researchers estimate that stress is a predisposing factor of fibromyalgia and, in fact, in most other diseases, in 80 percent of cases. Stress can cause the following symptoms and health problems, all of which are too familiar to people with fibromyalgia:

- Fatigue
- Headaches
- Insomnia or other changes in sleep patterns
- Memory loss
- Nightmares
- Mood changes or swings
- Prone to accidents
- Loss of enthusiasm and motivation to do anything
- Crying spells
- Lack of focus, inability to concentrate
- Gastrointestinal disorders
- Allergies
- Skin rashes or irritations
- Asthma
- Diarrhea or constipation
- Changes in appetite
- Teeth-grinding
- Cold hands
- Sweaty palms
- Shallow breathing
- Nervous twitches
- High blood pressure
- Lowered sexual drive
- Low self-esteem
- Depression

Stress has very definite physical effects. Almost all body organs and functions react to stress. When challenged or in a stressful situation, the brain prepares the body for defensive action—the fight-or-flight response—by releasing stress hormones, namely cortisol and adrenaline. These hormones raise the blood pressure and accelerate the heartbeat, as the body prepares to react to the situation (called the stressor). Digestion slows or stops, fats and sugars are released from stores in the body, cholesterol levels rise, and the muscles tense.

Over time, too much stress eventually inhibits the functioning of disease-fighting white blood cells and suppresses the immune response, leaving us susceptible to infection and disease. When the duration of the stress is sufficiently long, the body eventually enters a stage of exhaustion, as it cannot cope or adapt anymore.

To return to a state of balance and to rebuild strength, it is imperative to identify the cause of the stress and remove it from your diet or environment. Substances that most commonly cause a defensive reaction include:

- Wheat and gluten products
- Milk and dairy products
- Chocolate
- Sugar
- Alcohol
- Tea and coffee
- Smoking
- Grass pollens
- Fumes

Although most substances that trigger an adverse reaction usually produce an initial reaction within twenty-four hours, others have a long-term effect that shows up two or three days later. This can mean that the liver has exceeded its ability to rid itself of excess toxins. We will discuss ways in which to rejuvenate your liver and experience less fatigue and more energy, but first, let's look at some ways to manage stress.

Ways to Manage Stress

The type of effect stress has on you depends on how you handle it. Handling stress depends on being able to recognize it, knowing where it's coming from, and understanding your stress-management options, so you can choose the best one for your situation. While this might sound easy, it's not; knowing how to handle stress can take years to master, but it's never too late to start.

- Get regular exercise. Frequent exercise is probably one of the best physical stress-reduction techniques available. Exercise not only improves your overall health, it also helps you sleep. Another benefit of exercise is that it can cause the release of chemicals called endorphins, which give you a feeling of well-being and happiness.

- Practice deep breathing. It is a key element for calming yourself down. Take a few deep breaths and hold for a few seconds before letting them out slowly and gently. Repeat four or five times and you should feel more calm and relaxed.

- Try meditation. Many people find that regular meditation helps them to relax and handle stress. Meditation need not have spiritual or religious connotations. The idea behind meditation is to focus your thoughts on something relaxing for a sustained period of time. For example, you can meditate on a word such as "peace" or "relax." Or you might prefer to meditate on a pleasant scene or event. Meditation helps clear away toxins that have built up through stress or mental or physical activity. Try practicing it every day and you might find your approach to everything in your life is calming and steady.

- Eat a diet generous in whole foods, at least 50 percent of which should be raw foods. Fresh fruits and vegetables are loaded with vitamins, minerals, and phytonutrients, to help fight free radicals. Try eating a minimum of five to seven servings per day of vegetables, and notice how much calmer you feel.

- Stay away from processed and artificial foods, which only heap stress on the body. Avoid alcohol, sugar, caffeine, tobacco, and mood-altering drugs. These substances may offer temporary relief from stress, but they do nothing to resolve the problem and are harmful in the long term.

- Get plenty of rest each night. Nothing compares to the refreshment that a good night's sleep brings. The less sleep you get, the more stress will affect you, weakening your immune system and increasing the likelihood of your becoming ill. Try to be in bed early and be sure not to go to bed with a full stomach. Overnight is when your system does most of its repair and regenerative work. It should not direct energy toward digesting food—it should focus instead on restoring health and well-being.

Many other methods for dealing with stress are available. This list suggests some of the main ways you can achieve quick, positive results. Additional suggestions include avoiding drama and hassles; taking time off; pursuing a hobby; creating a stress-free home or work environment; experimenting with aromatherapy; and laughing more.

The Link with the Liver

The liver is the main detoxification organ, and its proper function is essential to a healthy immune system and our ability to fight disease. When the liver is overloaded with toxins or its detoxifying systems are compromised, the door is opened for chronic diseases such as fibromyalgia.

There are four basic reasons for poor liver function:

1. The presence of cumulative poisons. These include preservatives, alcohol, chemicals, insecticides, and other toxins that can accumulate in and impair the liver. Although a particular toxin may not build up in the liver, liver function may suffer if the functioning of other organs, especially the pancreas or kidneys, is adversely affected by the toxin.

2. An improper diet. A diet that is low in protein and high in carbohydrates and fats, especially hydrogenated fats and fried foods, is hard on the liver and might not provide sufficient

protein building blocks necessary for repair. Poor food choices include processed foods, junk foods, refined white flour products, white sugar products, and devitalized foods that have been robbed of natural vitamins, minerals, and enzymes.

3. Overeating. Overeating is one of the most common causes of liver malfunction. Overeating generates excess work for the liver, resulting in liver fatigue. The liver must detoxify the various chemicals present in our food supply, and when overworked, it may not detoxify harmful substances properly.

4. Drugs. Drugs put great strain on the liver's detoxification pathways. Drugs are unnatural to the body and cause the liver to work overtime to excrete these toxins. Often vitamin and mineral reserves are taken from elsewhere in the body to help the liver detoxify drugs and toxins. Excess alcohol also causes the liver to lose its functioning capacity, as does caffeine and oral contraceptives.

Sticking to a diet of nutrient-dense whole foods helps detoxify the liver and ensure its proper functioning.

Nutritional recommendations:

- Drink juice made from fresh, raw vegetables made daily with a juice-extracting machine. Juices made from carrots, cabbage, celery, garlic, kale, and beets all have incredible healing power.
- Avoid salt, which contributes to cellular imbalance and prevents detoxification.
- Avoid wheat and dairy, as these tend to slow detoxification.
- Avoid grapefruit, because it contains naringin, a flavonoid compound that gives grapefruit its characteristic bitter flavor and prevents liver detoxification.

- Avoid coffee, tea, alcohol, sugar in all forms, and artificial sweeteners.
- Adding alpha-lipoic acid, vitamin C, vitamin E, and B vitamins and bioflavonoids is highly beneficial.
- Herbs such as ginkgo biloba, dandelion, milk thistle (silymarin), and pycnogenol are highly beneficial.
- Minerals such as zinc and selenium are highly beneficial.

Try to consume the following every day:

- A large raw, green salad
- One serving of fresh seasonal fruit (apples, pears, blueberries)—not juice
- A minimum of three to four servings of lightly steamed green vegetables, such as broccoli, brussels sprouts, kale, collards, and cabbage
- A cup of cooked legumes, such as lentils or beans, or any other vegetable protein and/or a piece of lightly steamed or grilled fresh fish
- One cup (165 g) of whole-grain brown rice

Digestive Health and the Gluten-Free Diet

For people with fibromyalgia, choosing the right foods isn't easy. Food is a fairly contentious topic at the best of times. Many clients will tell me that they eat healthy and that they don't think their diet is tied to any of their symptoms. Upon closer inspection though, this is never the case and our diet is always the best starting place to examine when your goal is to get well. Symptoms of fatigue or brain fog nearly always have a nutritional component to them and a large percentage of the time food intolerance or allergies are the culprits behind them.

So, just how do you 1) choose the most nutritious foods to provide you with the best health possible, and 2) trust that you have chosen a healthy eating plan you can follow with confidence? A good starting point is that any diet-related advice should be based on sound scientific knowledge that is, in turn, based on an understanding of how the human body functions. While personal experiences or preferences, or the current fad diet or "miracle" product on the market, may make for interesting reading, it is definitely not the wisest way to choose a program for something as vitally important as your good health—especially when you're working on eliminating chronic pain, debilitating fatigue, and other fibromyalgia symptoms.

There are two key topics to investigate when you are determining the type of diet which is best suited for you. The first topic involves an understanding of the basic principles around food and diet that apply to all of us. For example, decades of scientific research have clearly shown that proper blood sugar control is an absolute requirement for maintaining proper body weight, good brain function, hormone balance, and to stimulate a healthy immune system. The second topic each of us must become familiar with is what specific foods are harmful and which foods are well-tolerated by our particular body chemistry. While we may do our best to follow what we believe is a healthy diet, we may be unwittingly causing ourselves problems by eating foods that are harmful to our individual genetic makeup.

Using nutrition and a thorough understanding of our digestive system as a starting point for reducing symptoms of fibromyalgia and attaining optimal health, we will review how a healthy digestive system functions. Then we will consider food intolerance and food allergies, with a particular focus on a newly discovered—and often misdiagnosed—condition referred to as sub-clinical gluten intolerance. Fortunately, sophisticated lab tests are now available that can screen for food intolerance and food allergies. These provide crucial information when it comes to determining what specific foods are right—or wrong—for you.

In my practice, I also use an adrenal stress profile to assess the levels of two important hormones produced by the adrenal glands: cortisol and DHEA. This profile reveals valuable information on how well clients have maintained blood sugar control over a period of time and, as such, is a key indicator of overall health. I also use gluten-free diets and metabolic/nutritional typing to evaluate clients' unique body chemistry and their bodies' reactions to what they eat and drink. Nutritional typing determines your individual nutritional requirements and dictates your body's response to what you eat and drink. For example, some people tend to be "protein" types and therefore require higher levels of protein throughout their day, while others may need higher ratios of carbohydrates for their metabolism to function optimally. Nutritional typing is a science that's based on your unique biochemistry, which makes it fairly accurate to evaluate your body's individual nutritional needs. More information about metabolic/nutritional typing is on page 54.

What follows provides a scientific starting point for you to begin making positive and sensible food choices. We'll start with a closer look at sub-clinical gluten intolerance and who is affected by this condition.

Sub-Clinical Gluten Intolerance and Who Does It Affect?

Sub-clinical gluten intolerance—sometimes referred to as "hidden" gluten intolerance—is a health problem at epidemic proportions in certain populations in the United States today. This is not a typical food allergy but an inherited condition, found most frequently in people with Irish, English, Scottish, Scandinavian and other Northern and Eastern European heritages. Researchers suspect that close to one in three Americans suffer from sub-clinical gluten intolerance. Since there are often no obvious symptoms, sub-clinical gluten intolerance frequently goes undetected or is misdiagnosed. This leaves many people to suffer the health consequences of this condition without ever realizing the true cause of their health woes.

Sub-clinical gluten intolerance was first documented in the United States by doctors who noticed their patients were struggling with chronic fatigue, weakened immune systems, and environmental illnesses. In 1994 a highly specialized salivary test for sub-clinical gluten intolerance paved the way for more comprehensive investigation into this condition. However, sub-clinical gluten intolerance still remains largely unrecognized by conventional medicine even though it has been well-documented in large groups of chronically ill patients.

Conventional medicine does recognize a more extreme form of this condition which is known as celiac disease. Celiac disease has overt symptoms such as disabling pain or blood in the stool, and the symptoms often begin with the introduction of glutinous foods in childhood. A blood test and biopsy of the small intestine can confirm the diagnosis. However, sub-clinical gluten intolerance remains largely undiagnosed and therefore many people continue to suffer its consequences. Symptoms can range from sudden or unexplained weight gain and fatigue, to achy joints and irritable bowel syndrome. Many people with fibromyalgia also suffer from sub-clinical gluten intolerance and probably aren't aware of it. Although not everyone is gluten-intolerant, everyone benefits from a two-month gluten-free diet because it forces us to eat less of the processed, refined foods that contain gluten, and eat more unprocessed foods such as organic vegetables, quality proteins, fats, and healthy carbohydrates. Later, I'll outline a gluten-free meal plan along with a list of foods to include in your diet and those to avoid.

Management of Sub-Clinical Gluten Intolerance

If your nutritionist has made a scientific diagnosis—for example, through an adrenal stress profile or nutritional typing—and determined that you have sub-clinical gluten intolerance, now what? Well, first you will want to know what foods contain gluten (or the gliadin molecule) so that you can avoid them. Wheat, rye, barley, kamut, spelt, teff, and couscous all contain gluten in varying concentrations and should be avoided. Some people are able to tolerate rice, corn, oats, buckwheat and millet as the glutens in these foods do not contain the gliadin molecule that can provoke an inflammatory response in the digestive tract. Quinoa and amaranth are usually "safe" as well. You will want to ensure that you do not have an allergy to any of these safe grains independent of your gluten sensitivity. A nutritionist can help you with this determination.

Soy

Approximately half of those sensitive to gluten are also intolerant to soy and soy products. If you are able to tolerate gliadin and do not have a soy allergy, then soybean products may be beneficial for you. Your nutritionist can advise you on what forms of soy to avoid and when it may be safe for you to integrate some soy products into your diet. For example, it is advisable to avoid all concentrated forms of soy protein such as soy protein powders, tofu, and tempeh when you are first eliminating gliadin from your diet.

On the safe list of foods are any type of meat, poultry; or fish; fruits, vegetables, and beans (with soybean products being a possible exception). As mentioned, rice, corn, buckwheat, and millet are okay unless you are allergic to them. Oats are generally okay, however, they are often processed in the same plants along with gluten products and may contain some cross contamination, thereby causing symptoms for some people.

A helpful supplement that can be used to assist your body's healing processes by further reducing inflammation and helping to protect irritated tissue is deglycerized licorice root. This herbal extract is available in most health food stores, and with the guidance of your nutritionist can be a useful aid to recovery from sub-clinical gluten intolerance.

A Healthy Digestive System

Good health requires proper digestion and absorption of nutrients from the foods we eat. Digestion begins when we chew our food, and digestive enzymes in our saliva begin to break it down. In our stomach, hydrochloric acid and pepsin further process our food, especially proteins. From here, our stomach contents enter our small intestine. While smaller in diameter than our large intestine, this remarkable organ is a crucial component of our digestive tract. The small intestine is covered with fingerlike protrusions called villi that increase the surface absorption area of the small intestine to be roughly the size of a basketball court! If these villi are irritated or damaged by a condition such as sub-clinical gluten intolerance, our ability to properly digest our food is negatively affected. Poorly digested food leads to poor absorption of the vital nutrients our body needs to maintain healthy function. In addition, tiny structures on the tips of the villi, called lacteals, can be destroyed by the body's reaction to gluten. As the lacteals are responsible for helping us absorb healthy fats, we are faced with a deficiency in fat-soluble nutrients such as vitamin A and vitamin E.

The lining of our small intestine, similar to our sinus passageways, lungs, mouth, and throat, is covered with a mucosal lining that acts as an important barrier to infectious organisms. In our small intestine this mucosal lining also has the vital function of absorption of nutrients for passage into our bloodstream. Under ongoing inflammatory stress like what we see with sub-clinical gluten intolerance, healthy mucosal tissue breaks down and allows molecules to pass into our blood stream that should not be there. This condition is known as intestinal permeability, more commonly called *leaky gut syndrome*. It can lead to a wide array of health problem, which includes indigestion, IBS, acid reflux, candida albicans, ulcers, food cravings, excess weight, and low hydrochloric acid production, to name a few.

Sub-Clinical Gluten Intolerance— What Is the Effect on Our Digestive Systems?

Once it has been determined that you have sub-clinical gluten intolerance, you will need to be patient and stay the course as it will take some time before you feel the benefits of your change in diet. It is not uncommon for it to take 60 days for inflammation to subside and from 9 to 12 months for the lining of the small intestine to heal. Some fortunate individuals begin to experience significant improvement within weeks of being on a gluten-free diet, while others may initially feel worse during the diet's early phases.

It is important to remember that for those of us with sub-clinical gluten intolerance, the 'wear and tear' on our digestive system has been ongoing for years. It just makes sense that it would take a few months for our bodies to repair and recover, and for us to experience a greater sense of well-being. Perhaps a closer look at just what happens to our digestive system if we have sub-clinical gluten intolerance will help us be patient and stick with our new improved eating patterns.

Inflammation of any part of our body is a familiar experience. If we are injured, our immune systems swing into high gear to fight the inflammation caused by the physical trauma or ensuing viral or bacterial infection. In sub-clinical gluten intolerance, the gliadin molecule causes an inflammatory reaction when it comes into contact with the wall of the small intestine. This low-level wear and tear may go on for years as the tissue lining the small intestine gradually becomes damaged. The initial reaction to the gliadin (gluten) is heat, redness, swelling and a disruption of the normal function of the small intestine. Blood vessels react to combat the inflammation, and within 12 to 14 hours the body's response fades, only to reactivate the next time gluten makes its appearance. With a regular diet of gluten-containing grains, it's not hard to picture the long-term effects of repeated inflammation on our small intestine and other body systems.

In addition to the actual harm done to the lining of our intestines in sub-clinical gluten intolerance, a key function of our digestive system—to absorb nutrients from our diet—is seriously hampered. This poor absorption and failure to deliver nutrients has a negative impact on several of our body systems.

Immune and Hormonal Systems Negatively Affected

If our digestive system is compromised, other important body systems are negatively impacted as well and this is very often the case with fibromyalgia syndrome. Two of these systems are our immune system and our hormonal system. Misdiagnoses can occur if the root cause, which is often sub-clinical gluten intolerance, is not understood to be at the base of the problem

Specialized immune system cells—called immunocytes—line our small intestine. These cells produce secretory IgA, an important component of the mucous lining that is a first-line immune system defense. The inflammation that occurs in individuals with sub-clinical gluten intolerance can destroy these cells with the result of opening the door to intestinal infections by parasites, bacteria, viruses, yeast, or fungal infections.

A weakened IgA secretion can also disturb our body's ability to process food antigens, which can create significant health problems. Antigens, substances that are foreign to the human body—such as food—all have a marker that the body recognizes as safe or unsafe. For example, a virus that causes the common cold has an antigen marker that our body will recognize and then go to work concocting antibodies to destroy that virus. Typically, we don't react to food antigens,

but a weakening of our small intestines' immune defense system can lead to overreaction to food antigens, which in turn leads to more stress on our digestive system.

Any stress that inflames the digestive tract—and sub-clinical gluten intolerance is certainly a stressor— triggers our body to create corticosteroids, mostly in the form of the hormone cortisol. Many people are familiar with corticosteroid medications such as prednisone or cortisone. This overproduction of cortisol suppresses our immune system function and works against our general good health. Abnormal cortisol production negatively affects our hormonal and immune systems. Elevated cortisol suppresses our immune responses while also causing a catabolic/breakdown state to exist in our body, which leads to adrenal insufficiency. Eventually we suffer the symptoms of adrenal exhaustion such as fatigue, depression, loss of libido, allergies, and frequent illness.

When our digestive system is under chronic inflammatory stress, our healthy mucosal small intestine lining begins to break down and cause a condition called increased permeability, also known as leaky gut syndrome. Leaky gut syndrome is similar to a screen door with large holes in it: unwanted insects just fly on through! In the case of our bodies, molecules that were never intended to have access to our bloodstream can now gain entry. Our immune system struggles under further stress as it tries to cope with these intruders.

Nutritional Deficiencies

The lack of normal absorption in the small intestine leads to nutritional deficiencies; this comes as no surprise! We've already seen how the loss of fat-soluble nutrients leads to essential fatty acid deficiencies, including vitamin A and vitamin E. The negative spin-off effect is immense because these nutrients are critical for the optimal functioning of every cell in our bodies. Many processes, including blood sugar control, nerve cell function, steroid hormone production and anti-oxidant formation are reliant on fat-soluble nutrients to do their work. This includes the production of our reproductive hormones and adrenal hormones including estrogen, testosterone, progesterone, cortisol, and DHEA, and can disrupt the normal menstrual cycle.

In addition, poor calcium absorption coupled with abnormal corticosteroid production hastens osteoporosis (brittle bones). Deficiencies in iron, B12 and folic acid can lead to fatigue, mild depression, memory loss and a greater risk for elevated homocysteine levels which are a key factor in the development of heart disease. Amino acids—the building blocks of our bodies—are vital for the production of neurotransmitters such as serotonin, which is important for elevating moods and lowering depression. If you are unable to digest protein well or cannot absorb the amino acids from protein, over time you will develop deficiencies that ultimately affect brain chemistry, function and other body processes. A nutritional approach which looks at your protein intake, along with your body's ability to digest it and absorb its nutrients, can provide a pathway for greater health and wellbeing. For some people with food sensitivities, this one factor can prevent recovery from weight gain, and lead to fatigue, recurrent infections and an unhappy cycle of chronic illness!

Food Allergies and Intolerances

Most of us have heard of lactose intolerance. This is the body's inability to digest the carbohydrate portion of milk products. What isn't as widely known is that lactose intolerance frequently accompanies gluten intolerance. Lactase, a specialized enzyme that aids digestion of lactose in milk, is usually lacking in people with sub-clinical gluten intolerance, as is the sucrase enzyme that breaks down sugar or sucrose. This leads to problems in digesting pasteurized dairy products such as cheese and ice cream. Plus, pasteurization and homogenization destroys the enzymes in milk that help us digest it, the healthy bacteria in milk that

help keep the gut working well, and the beneficial fats in dairy, rendering what could be a very nurturing and healing foods a potentially harmful product.

People with sub-clinical gluten intolerance need to avoid pasteurized cows' milk products, especially in the first two months of eliminating gluten from their diet. Some people may be able to gradually tolerate raw or unpasteurized dairy products again in nine months to a year, although some people retain a permanent sensitivity to dairy products. Your nutritionist can provide helpful advice to you on this matter.

Sub-clinical gluten intolerance often leads to the development of multiple delayed food allergies due to leaky gut syndrome. What this means is that foods that would otherwise be tolerated become allergenic, and you are no longer able to eat them without symptoms occurring. Such a response, as noted, involves the inappropriate launching of an immune attack upon undigested or partially digested food particles that have entered the blood stream due to increased permeability of the intestinal lining. This maladaptive response to food or food components is thought to be autoimmune in nature. Symptoms can range from extreme fatigue and chronic pain, to skin eruptions or insomnia. With the guidance of your nutritionist, a food rotation diet or further food allergy testing may be good routes to try to determine delayed food allergies. It is important to note than many people who are gluten intolerant do not test positive on food allergy testing for wheat, rye, barley, and other gluten-containing grains. Regardless of the result of this allergy testing, it is still critical to avoid gluten-containing foods if you are gluten intolerant as intestinal damage is still taking place.

To complicate the picture a little more, food cravings often accompany gluten intolerance. Strangely enough, it has frequently been observed that people crave what they are allergic to! It cannot be overstressed that if you crave gluten, this indicates a high probability that you are gluten sensitive. You can pick up a free copy of my Symptoms Blueprint on my website at www.FoodsforFibromyalgia.com to help you determine which foods may be causing you symptoms.

List of Gluten-Free Foods to Include
Protein
It is very important to eat adequate amounts of protein at each meal. The amino acids in protein foods are instrumental in forming cells, repairing tissue, making antibodies, carrying oxygen throughout the body, assisting muscle activity, increasing neurotransmitter production, as well as being part of the hormonal system. The variety of protein sources and the quality are important. It is best to try and limit protein consumption to sources that are organic, hormone-free, free-range, grass-fed, and "wild" in the case of fish. Canned salmon or tuna is generally safe as it's usually canned right on the dock with fresh fish that's been caught in the wild. Use only fresh meats: avoid those that are processed and packaged as they contain sulfites or sulfates and can be especially harmful to people with fibromyalgia. It is important to divide the day's total protein over the course of the day. You may need to increase this amount if you are a protein type.

Choose from these sources:

Beef, pork, and lamb: Eat up to four times a week.

Fish: Eat a variety of grilled, steamed, baked, or poached, but do not bread or deep-fry. Choose wild over farm-raised.

Poultry: Eat a variety of chicken, turkey, and Cornish game hen, in a mix of dark and white meat. Do not bread or deep-fry. Acceptable cooking methods are grilled, steamed, baked, or roasted.

Eggs: Eat as often as three times a week. The yolk contains nutrients that denature when cooked through, so when you can, eat eggs that are soft-boiled, sunny side up, or over-easy.

Nuts: These may be used as a protein snack source. Raw and organic tree nuts are preferable.

Cheese: All cows' milk products must be eliminated for the first two weeks. Choose goat and sheep cheeses and goats' milk yogurt as alternatives if your specific plan allows. After two weeks, you may introduce raw (unpasteurized) dairy into your diet.

Carbohydrates
Carbohydrates include fruits, grains, beans, and vegetables. The best carbohydrates are plant-based, nutrient dense, and rich in vitamins.

Vegetables
Nutrient-dense vegetables provide an abundance of the vitamins and minerals that sustain your body. Again, quality and variety are key. Your body is best nourished by high-quality organic produce. Many therapeutic nutrients such as antioxidants and flavonoids are associated with the properties that give vegetables their color, so make sure you are eating a good range. Eating vegetables raw or lightly cooked helps maintain vitamin content and makes them easier to digest.

Green vegetables: Eat an abundance of greens. They are high in essential minerals and low in calories. Good examples include kale, collard greens, spinach, swiss chard, bok choy, brussels sprouts, and salad greens. Dark-green steamed vegetables are superior to salad greens.

Orange and yellow vegetables: Eat these in smaller portions and always balance with green vegetables and protein. Some examples include yams, winter squash, and carrots.

Onions and garlic are high in sulphur which cleanses the liver. Eat these as desired, unless allergic.

Fruits

Fresh, whole fruits are allowed in moderation. Fruits tend to be high in sugar, which ferments in your gut and can feed harmful pathogens such as candida. Your best fruit choices include berries: raspberries, strawberries, and blueberries. Other fruits to include are apples, grapefruit, and pears. Avoid bananas and grapes because they are higher on the glycemic index and can wreak havoc with your blood sugar, as will dried fruit, which may also contain harmful preservatives.

Beans

Beans and legumes are an excellent source of carbohydrate and do contain some amino acids, which are building blocks of protein. They can be eaten frequently as part of your balanced diet.

Grains

Only gluten-free grains are permitted. Acceptable grains include quinoa, buckwheat, amaranth, arrowroot, millet, corn, and white or brown rice. Potatoes are acceptable unless you are sensitive to nightshade vegetables (which are tomatoes, potatoes, peppers, and eggplant) and should be avoided in this case. There are now rice breads and millet breads available for toast and sandwiches, as well as rice-corn-, and quinoa-based pastas. Check with your local grocery store and ask them to get them in for you if you are not able to find them.

Fats

It is important to have some healthy fat at each meal. Fats are an excellent source of fuel for your body and they also have no effect on your insulin levels making them quite stable as an energy source. As with all food groups, it is important to give your body variety. Choose from extra-virgin cold-pressed olive oil, coconut, walnut, sesame, and real butter. Raw butter is ideal because it possesses healing qualities. Ghee, which is clarified butter, is the safest and most healthful. Avoid all margarines, hydrogenated and partially hydrogenated oils, as well as canola oil and processed mayonnaise. Grape-seed oil is stable for cooking at high temperatures as is coconut oil. Olive oil is not as stable at high temperatures unless you add a little water to the pan first when using in stir-fries.

Beverages

Water is still the best beverage to drink. Our bodies are seventy percent water, and it is considered a nutrient, optimizing digestive function and elimination of toxins from your body. Always choose filtered or pure spring water. It's best to avoid fruit juices, caffeine, and alcoholic beverages, especially beer, which contains gluten. If you are a daily caffeine consumer, try switching to more natural sources such as green tea, which is also high in antioxidants.

Snack Suggestions

Include two or three healthy snacks in your daily food plan. Never let your blood sugar dip too low or go for more than about two or three hours without eating. Try eating several smaller meals throughout your day and take some snacks with you when you are traveling or on the road. Snack suggestions can include the following:

- Hardboiled or deviled eggs, along with half to one cup of vegetables
- 1 to 2 ounce piece of chicken, turkey, fish, beef, or lamb, along with half to one cup of vegetables
- One to two ounces goat or sheep cheese, and half to one cup of vegetables
- One piece fruit and small handful of nuts, or 1 tablespoon nut or seed butter
- Half cup of sunflower seeds, pumpkin seeds

- Raw nuts, 6–10 nuts per snack. Choose from almonds (higher in protein content), walnuts, brazil nuts, and pecans. Raw and organic nuts containing enzymes are preferred. Be sure to chew all nuts thoroughly or grind them up and add them to a smoothie.
- Protein shake or smoothie (add one cup fresh berries and handful of fresh raw spinach).
- Gluten-free muffin with added nuts and berries (see recipes).
- One quarter of fresh avocado on rice crackers.
- Nut butters such as almond or tahini (sesame seed butter) at 1 tablespoon per snack.
- It's best to avoid peanuts for a minimum of three to four weeks as they are a potential allergen and more difficult to digest.
- Cashews, pistachios, and macadamia nuts are higher in fat content and best left out until weight and food cravings are properly managed.

Sample Meal Plans
Breakfast
Eat a nutrient-dense breakfast that includes protein. Never skip breakfast. Studies show that people who eat a solid, healthy, balanced breakfast are healthier, have fewer food cravings throughout their day and make wiser food choices. In addition, eating a healthy breakfast will ensure you have fewer symptoms and a lot more energy throughout your day.

- Dinner leftovers—include meats such as turkey, chicken, fish with vegetables and salad
- Eggs—poached or over-easy are preferable cooking methods. Eat with sautéed vegetables or mixed spinach or lettuce greens.
- Sauté veggies (onions, spinach, tomatoes, rosemary, basil, etc.) in coconut or olive oil, push to the side of the pan and proceed to cook the eggs in the vegetable oil/juice sauces.

- Add rice, yams, and sweet potatoes as appropriate for your specific food plan and always balance with the protein and vegetables.
- Omelets—add lots of sautéed veggies, avocado, salsa, and feta or goat cheese if allowed on your specific diet plan. Be creative! Enjoy with chicken or turkey sausage.
- Turkey, chicken, lamb sausages—with sautéed vegetables, rice/lentils/beans/yams (as appropriate for you).
- Protein smoothie—include fresh raw veggies (kale, spinach, swiss chard), and a cup of berries. Add a raw egg to increase protein content.

Lunch
- Dinner leftovers—include meats such as turkey, chicken, fish, lamb, and beef with vegetables and/or salad. Include a serving of rice/beans/lentils/yams.
- Raw salad with turkey, chicken, eggs, tuna, salmon, beef, lamb, or sausages. Use balsamic-olive oil dressing, or any olive oil based dressing. (Make your own dressing—see recipes).
- Turkey, chicken, fish, lamb, beef, with sautéed vegetables or salad. Include a serving of rice/beans/lentils/yam.
- Omelets with vegetables, feta or goat cheese if allowed on your specific food plan. Include a serving of rice/beans/lentils/yam.
- Wraps (gluten-free)— include chicken, turkey, or fish, with vegetables and/or salad.
- Soup and salad—include beans, lentils, and meats.

Dinner
- Turkey, chicken, beef, seafood, lamb—marinated, grilled, steamed, poached, herbed, spiced, or baked, with salad, vegetables and appropriate portions of rice/beans/lentils/yams.
- Soup and salad—include beans, lentils, and meats.
- Example: turkey meatloaf served with steamed broccoli, cauliflower, kale, and brown rice.

Eating Out at Restaurants

- Meat, turkey, chicken, fish, lamb—grilled, poached, steamed, or stir-fried, with salad, vegetables and appropriate portions of rice/beans/lentils/yams.
- Ask for substitutions of vegetables or salads in place of starches (such as potatoes or pasta)
- Make it easy on yourself—ask them to hold the bread basket.
- Ask if your menu choice has any hidden flours.
- Rice bowls or rice noodles (protein, vegetables, and rice) save for evening meal.
- The Bunless Burger—ask for protein wrapped in lettuce.

Hidden Glutens

Read food labels carefully. Glutens can be hidden under such names as hydrolyzed vegetable protein, modified food starch, dextrin, and natural flavorings. Gluten may also be found in the alcohol used in flavorings such as vanilla, and in distilled vinegar and veined cheese such as blue cheese and roquefort. Even the tiniest amount could be enough to keep you from feeling the best that you can.

Intolerable Foods/Drinks	Tolerable Foods/ Drinks	
Wheat	Rice	Tapioca
Rye	Wild Rice	Taro
Soy	Corn	Bean Flours
Spelt	Buckwheat	Coconut Flours
Barley	Millet	Barley Grass & Barley Malt
Kamut	Quinoa	Wheat Grass
Triticale	Amaranth	Vinegars
Teff	Oats (organic)	
Couscous	Arrowroot	

Gluten-Free Diet Guidelines:

Use these guidelines when you're shopping. Post a copy of them up on your refrigerator or kitchen wall to help you become more familiar with the foods that are most compatible for your new eating plan.

	Foods to Enjoy	Comments	Foods to Avoid
Protein Choose organic/free range/ hormone free	Beef, lamb, poultry (chicken, turkey, game hen), fish	Red meats: grass fed Poultry: eat both dark & white meats Fish: choose wild over farmed Eggs: free range	Fruits, vegetables, grains
Carbohydrate vegetables Organic where possible	Dark leafy greens: swiss chard, kale, mustard greens, spinach, onions, root vegetables	Eating vegetables raw or lightly cooked helps maintain vitamin & mineral content	Canned vegetables
Carbohydrate fruits Organic where possible	Whole, fresh fruits in moderation Best choices: berries, apples, grapefruit	Choose seasonal, local fruits	Avoid bananas, grapes, and dried fruits as they tend to spike blood sugar
Carbohydrate grains Organic where possible	White/brown rice, beans & legumes, corn, potato, oats, amaranth, buchwheat, millet, and quinoa are also fine	Bread & pasta made from non-gluten flours are available	White flour, wheat flour, spelt, barley, rye, kamut, teff. Avoid refined carbs such as sugar and corn syrup
Fats/Oils Organic where possible	Extra virgin olive oil, sesame oil, coconut oil, real organic butter, ghee, avocado, flaxseed oil	Include good fats/oils with each meal. Supplement with fish oils (omega-3)	Margarines, hydrogenated & partially hydrogenated oils, canola, processed mayonnaise
Drinks	Filtered water, herbal teas	Water is the best beverage to drink; it helps to optimize digestive function & elimination	Caffeine, fruit juices, beer (contains gluten)
Superfoods	Spices: garlic, ginger, cinnamon, turmeric, sea vegetables	Use as an accompaniment to meals	Choose spices that have not been irradiated

Opportunistic Infections

The structural changes to the small intestine from gluten intolerance create a perfect habitat for the development of pathogenic infections such as parasites. The lengthening of these structures—called crypts—creates deep pockets where parasites can hide out from our immune system and thrive. As inflammation caused by sub-clinical gluten intolerance also damages our immune cells, parasitic infections can take hold and become chronic.

Candida (yeast) is another opportunistic "bug" that can take advantage of a digestive tract weakened by sub-clinical gluten intolerance. Candida overgrowth can become invasive and cause a host of digestive disturbances. It is often a most difficult condition to diagnose because it can affect each sufferer in a different way. Many doctors are unfamiliar with candida and its relationship toward many other conditions, thereby missing an important piece of the healing process. For this reason, candida is often misdiagnosed and the symptoms are treated instead of the underlying cause. Some studies have shown that greater than 70 percent of fibromyalgia patients have a mycoplasma or fungal infection component to their disease. Symptoms of candida (a fungus) include:

- Fatigue or lethargy
- Feelings of being drained
- Poor memory
- Inability to concentrate
- Brain fog
- Muscle aches
- Muscle weakness or paralysis
- Pain and/or swelling in joints
- Abdominal pain
- Insomnia
- Anxiety attacks or crying
- Bloating, belching or intestinal gas
- Numbness, burning or tingling
- Cold hands or feet and/or chilliness
- Shaking or irritable when hungry
- Headaches
- Food sensitivity or intolerance

Although researchers are now developing lab tests on blood and feces to diagnose fungal and yeast-related conditions, the primary methods used to date have been a medical history, questionnaire, and response to treatment. Practically, patients with candida often have to diagnose themselves because the symptoms are so widespread and confusing. The consensus is that many more people are suffering from candida than those few who are diagnosed correctly. You will find a full questionnaire to help you assess yourself on my website www.foodsforfibromyagalia.com.

Food as Medicine

It bears repeating that food is the ultimate medicine for achieving good health. There is no drug, vitamin pill, herb, or nutritional supplement that can influence your health quite as profoundly as your diet. Our nutritional requirements change throughout our lives, so it's important to fine-tune your dietary needs. Fine-tuning your diet from time to time is essential, because your metabolism is subject to occasional shifts. When you pay attention to—and learn to interpret—the multiple messages your body continuously transmits, a change will occur, and you will find yourself naturally selecting the foods that your body needs.

Food is a major determinant of health that is directly under our control. We cannot always control pollution, heredity, noise, environment, and the social and emotional behaviors of others, but we can certainly choose what to and what not to eat. Food is utilized throughout the day for sustenance and energy—consequently, it has enormous influence on the health of the body and mind. Food has been used as an essential part of medicine and to prevent disease for centuries. It's up to each of us to pay close attention to the principles of food as medicine and choose wisely for our health.

When we work consistently on a wellness lifestyle, particularly in the area of daily food and nutrition, disease will fade away and you will not succumb to the latest bug that's going around. You can expect to be healthier in ten years than you are today.

Of course, we age and we may meet with an unexpected illness, but in general, people who pay attention to what they eat and how they feel have a greater sense of well-being and resistance to disease. They also feel more responsible and in control of their lives. We all want to feel as young as possible. We want to enjoy vibrant health all the days of our life. When you apply the methods and principles described in this book, these desires move beyond something merely to wish for, toward something entirely attainable.

The Will to Change

Research has shown that hundreds of people have systematically and effectively reversed their fibromyalgia. One way in which we bring about health and healing in ourselves is by becoming more aware of what we are doing to create our ill health. Once we recognize that the foods we eat can have either a negative or positive impact on our health, we will want to eat in a way that enables the body to heal itself. We can heal ourselves simply by changing the environment inside our bodies. Potentially harmful invaders will have nowhere to grow and will be rendered harmless.

The reward for being willing to experiment and make changes can be profound: You will gain the confidence that your body will function smoothly and effortlessly into advanced age. And when and if it doesn't? Then it's back to the drawing board. Life is all about change, and every symptom has a lesson to teach.

The good news is that the human body is a self-regenerating organism. According to Dr. Deepak Chopra, author of *Quantum Healing*, we replace 98 percent of all our cells inside of a single year.

He writes, "98 percent of the 100 trillion cells that made up our body last year are no longer there."

- Every six months: new bones
- Every ten days: a new stomach lining
- Every three months: new blood cells

In one year, we can rebuild our blood, our cells, our organs, and in turn our immunity. Change the quality of nutrients we give the body, and we can literally recreate ourselves from the inside out.

We start by telling ourselves that we are worth whatever it takes to achieve this goal and that we have the will to change and to make choices that support our health and well-being. One of the first steps is to reverse the conditions that brought about our health problems in the first place and to note the choices we make (or fail to make) on a daily basis. We begin by taking more time to nourish ourselves with healing foods that provide the nutrients and other substances our body needs to function optimally. We do this by choosing those foods that support this healing and eliminating those that don't.

We must focus on health, rather than convenience, and develop better eating habits to bring about optimum good health. Instead of asking if a particular food looks and tastes good, we should ask: Is this food healthful, will it contribute to my biochemical balance, help me feel better, and finally, will it taste good? We need to exercise regularly and think positive thoughts. We need to relax alone and with friends and find ways to reduce the stress in our lives. We need to respect and look after our body's systems, and we need to create balance. This requires a serious commitment.

Summary

As we have seen, untreated sub-clinical gluten intolerance can create a range of health problems beyond damage to our digestive system. Our immune system and our hormonal system are also negatively affected by this condition. Left unchecked, sub-clinical gluten intolerance promotes a negative series of events in our bodies which can leave us feeling in poor health. Fortunately, scientific testing procedures such as the adrenal stress profile can point us towards the origin of these problems. By implementing changes to our diet which take into account our unique needs, we can get on the road to optimal health and well-being.

For most people, most of the time, the answer to health problems will not come from drugs. In the main, safest, most effective, speedy, and affordable solutions come from lifestyle choices—specifically, the air we breathe, the water we drink, and the food we eat. There is considerable proof that good food, air, and water lead to good sleep, good thoughts, and ultimately to balance and good health. Fibromyalgia is treatable, and the treatment consists of modifying our diet and environment.

To overcome fibromyalgia you need a holistic strategy with sound nutrition and healthy lifestyle adjustments.

- Taking medications and drugs often leads to a cascade of adverse reactions and side effects that further diminish health.
- What is needed most is to change the way you live and to live in harmony with your genes, by eating foods and nutrients that nourish and strengthen, rather than upset, your body's biochemistry.
- When your body is providing you with symptoms, or when you've been diagnosed with a chronic disorder, you must choose to make definite changes to your lifestyle.
- Researchers estimate that stress triggers fibromyalgia in 80 percent of cases.
- Too much stress over time will eventually suppress the immune response and leave us susceptible to infection and disease.

- To return to a state of balance and to rebuild strength, it is imperative to identify the cause of stress and remove it from your diet or environment.
- Stress can be managed simply through regular exercise, deep breathing, meditation, ample rest, and a proper diet.
- The liver is the main detoxification organ, and its proper function is essential to a healthy immune system and our ability to fight disease.
- There are four basic reasons for poor liver function: the presence of cumulative poisons, an improper diet, overeating, and drugs.
- Sticking to a diet of nutrient-dense whole foods is best, because these foods help detoxify the liver and ensure that it functions properly.
- To overcome fibromyalgia, we need to focus on health, rather than convenience, and develop better eating habits, exercise regularly, think positive thoughts, relax to reduce stress, look after our body's systems, and create balance.
- Sub-clinical gluten intolerance affects millions of people and causes many symptoms associated with fibromyalgia.
- Gluten intolerance leads to adrenal deficiency which affects two important hormones: cortisol and DHEA. An Adrenal Stress Profile test will you help determine this.
- People with sub-clinical gluten intolerance usually do best when they avoid pasteurized cows' milk products, and soy products.

CHAPTER 4

FOCUSING ON COLORFUL NUTRITION: WE ARE WHAT WE EAT

Changing our eating and lifestyle habits is crucial to overcoming fibromyalgia, and it requires a firm will and commitment. It is particularly important to alter or eliminate the environmental conditions that produced fibromyalgia and to effectively rebalance the body's biochemistry. In these days of fast foods, sticking to a properly balanced diet can be challenging, but the changes are well worth the effort and will quickly translate to increased vitality and energy and reduced chronic symptoms. Now that we have decided to improve our diet as a chief element in overcoming fibromyalgia, we'll look at its necessary nutritional components. We'll also see how these components combine holistically to create a pathway to vibrant health and wellness.

If we are to become healthy and rid our body of sickness, we must give the body what it needs by way of proper nourishment and fuel. But first, we need to learn what these fuels are and how to administer them. The purpose of this chapter is to teach you just that.

Cells and Energy

Every biochemical process in your body is entirely dependent on the rate, quality, and amount of available energy. As you may already know, *metabolism* is simply the total of all the chemical and biological activities necessary to sustain life. Metabolic life functions are many and diverse and can be summarized as nutrition, transport, respiration, synthesis, regulation, growth, and reproduction. These metabolic activities require energy to run our bodies and sustain life, and we acquire them from air, water, sunlight, and food (nutrients). The raw materials in the foods we eat (vitamins, minerals, enzymes, and others) are particularly important, because they're used by our bodies to repair, rebuild, and heal tissue. Foods and nutrients also provide the fuel that is oxidized (or burned) in our cells to provide energy for our metabolic activities. It is on the cellular level that all metabolic activity takes place and where efficiency or inefficiency is determined.

The overall lack of energy and constant fatigue that characterizes fibromyalgia is not such a mystery when looked at from a nutrition perspective. Fibromyalgia is a symptom of biochemical imbalances, and these biochemicals affect the whole body. Fad diets and diets consisting largely of refined and processed foods, alcohol, caffeine, and toxic elements can easily lead to a biochemical imbalance. Even the nutrient content of a "healthy" diet can be inadequate, depending on the soil in which the food was grown and the method in which it was prepared.

Minerals provide the foundation for countless metabolic functions and are the basis of human nutrition, upon which all other nutrients are based. It is absolutely vital that we eat a properly balanced diet that furnishes us with our daily supply of minerals. There are seven macrominerals—calcium, magnesium, potassium, sodium, sulphur, phosphorus, and chloride—which we need in minute amounts but whose absence results in many disease conditions. More than thirty trace minerals are known to be essential to life. These include iron, iodine, boron, manganese, zinc, copper, and chromium. Minerals are readily supplied from sources such as fresh fruits and vegetables, whole grains, raw nuts, and seeds. These minerals are important, especially in proper ratios, because they provide us with balance and health. However, mineral balance can also become upset, in a variety of ways.

Common Causes of Mineral Imbalances

- Improper nutritional intake. High levels of processed foods, caffeine, chemicals and preservatives, and alcohol, as well as fad diets can lead to a biochemical imbalance.
- Medication. Both prescription and over-the-counter medications can deplete the body's stores of nutrient minerals and increase levels of toxic metals. Examples include oral contraceptives, antacids, and diuretics.
- Stress. Physical and emotional stress can deplete the body of many nutrients and reduce its ability to absorb and utilize them.
- Pollution and environmental toxins. We are continually exposed to a variety of toxin sources, such as cigarettes, fossil fuels, hair dyes, dental amalgams, hydrogenated oils, antiperspirants, lead-based cosmetics, and pesticides.

- Inherited patterns. We may inherit a genetic predisposition toward mineral imbalances that can result in deficiencies and excesses.
- Soil conditions. Much of the soil in which our food grows has been depleted of vital minerals, in turn reducing our body's supplies of mineral nutrients.
- Nutritional supplements. Taking improper amounts or an incorrect type of nutritional supplements can contribute to a biochemical imbalance.

Our health is constantly being helped or hurt at the cellular level, and trace minerals are at the heart of this. If you have fibromyalgia, something—or more likely several things—has gone wrong. It's up to you to make the necessary changes, and to do this, you need to understand how you are supposed to function as a healthy and vital being. Our very life force stems from our cells, and when we select foods that nourish us on a cellular level, they generate the energy we need to keep going. Deep in every cell are tiny energy-producing "factories" called mitochondria. Many fibromyalgia abnormalities can be related to abnormal mitochondria. One study demonstrated that patients with fibromyalgia tend to have low levels of adenosine triphosphate (ATP), a molecule essential for storing and transporting energy within the cells of all living organisms.

The system malfunctions or breaks down because of an insufficient fuel supply, such as necessary trace minerals and vitamins, or because these energy factories have become polluted from too many toxins and chemicals. This leads to fatigue. In an effort to boost energy levels, typically a medication is prescribed, resulting in a further upset of the delicate balance between our cells and our metabolism. Medication may be a good short-term symptom reliever, but it does not address the cause of the problem. It can also restrict your ability to digest foods and impair absorption of nutrients, thereby adding to your symptoms. What the body needs is proper sources and supplies of fuel, which must come from the food we eat and the nutrition the food contains. We need to be educated about what the proper fuel sources are.

Let's take a look at the fuels the body requires to restore its balance and to function optimally.

Energizing the Body with the Right Fuels

Preventive medicine starts with what you put into your body: the food you eat, the air you breathe, and the water you drink. Our health is always being challenged, whether by the neighbor's cold or exhaust fumes in traffic. What we take into our body—healthy food, drugs, clean water, or junk food—can dramatically affect our ability to stay healthy. Because many people with fibromyalgia have many sensitivities, to various foods, to chemicals, and environmental pollutants, it's important that they avoid as many of them as possible. Researchers from the University of Florida who studied fibromyalgia patients concluded that food intolerance and certain chemicals added to foods led to significant exacerbation of symptoms including pain, swelling, and joint stiffness.

To a large extent, your nutritional status determines your capacity to maintain health and energy levels and your ability to adapt to your environment. If your environment is too hostile (excessive junk food, contaminated air and water, for example), you cannot adapt and disease ensues. If your environment is nourishing, you build up a greater resistance to disease and are more likely to experience health and vitality. It is equally important to reduce or remove toxic substances in the body, such as anti-nutrients and environmental chemicals and pollutants.

Whole Foods: Organic, Raw and Live Produce

The most important foundation for health is to eat foods that provide the energy and nutrients required to keep the body in perfect balance. A good deal of energy is consumed and wasted by the body's attempts to disarm or rid the body of toxic chemicals from our food sources. The toxins that cannot be eliminated accumulate in body tissue and contribute to conditions such as fibromyalgia. Unfortunately, it is virtually impossible to avoid these substances completely, because there is nowhere on our planet that is not somehow contaminated by the products of our modern chemical age. We must therefore be diligent in making the wisest choices possible.

Choosing organic foods whenever possible is the nearest we can get to eating a pure diet. The healthiest fruits and vegetables are those that have been grown organically—without the pesticides, herbicides, artificial fertilizers, and growth-stimulating chemicals that are potentially toxic to our bodies. Raw organic food is the most natural and beneficial way to take food into the body. Raw (also called live) foods also contain enzymes that help digest food more completely, allowing for the increased absorption and assimilation of vital nutrients within the food. Cooking food at temperatures above 118°F (48°C) destroys enzymes and limits the uptake of nutrients. Try to ensure that at least 50 percent of your fresh produce intake is in its raw state in salads and other dishes. If raw produce does not agree with you because of weak digestion capabilities, lightly steam your vegetables until just tender.

For people suffering from rheumatic disorders and fibromyalgia, studies have shown that a diet comprising whole foods brings the body back to a state of health and dramatically improves symptoms. In addition to the fact that whole foods are high in antioxidants, which possess anti-inflammatory properties, there are other factors, such as fiber and essential fatty acids found in whole unadulterated foods, that function together to increase immunity and improve overall health.

Most fruits and vegetables should be eaten in their entirety, because every part, including the skin, contains valuable nutrients. Eat at least eight to ten servings of colorful fruits and vegetables a day. That may sound like a lot, but one serving is only half a cup, and this food source is crucial to winning the battle against fibromyalgia. These plant foods are the greatest source of the vitamins, minerals, antioxidants, and phytonutrients (see next section) that help create and preserve health. Everyone—from physicians and scientists to health experts—agrees that eating fruits and vegetables is paramount to enjoying longevity, energy, and lasting health.

Phytonutrients—Nature's Pharmacy

The term *phyto* originates from a Greek word meaning "plant." Phytonutrients are the biologically active substances in plants that are responsible for giving them color, flavor, and natural disease resistance. In the last couple of decades, scientists have begun to see that they provide a vital biological function in humans, as well. Fruits, vegetables, grains, legumes, nuts, and teas are the richest sources of phytonutrients. Unlike traditional nutrients, such as proteins, fats, and carbohydrates, and vitamins and minerals, phytonutrients are not essential for life, but they help your body work optimally. Some people prefer the term *phytochemicals.*

Several studies examining the role of vegetarian and vegan diets (which are loaded with phytonutrients) in treating fibromyalgia have reported positive results. A study in 2000 looked at the potential role of antioxidants from a vegan diet in people with fibromyalgia and found significant increases in general health and reduced pain and stiffness. In another study, carried out with fibromyalgia

patients by the University of Finland, researchers examined a raw (or living) foods vegan diet consisting of fruits, vegetables, seeds, sprouts, and nuts (all foods containing high levels of phytonutrients). The results showed that fibromyalgia patients whose diets had the highest levels of serum carotenoids (lutein, lycopene, alpha carotene, and beta carotene) and flavonoids (quercetin and hesperidin), reported significant improvements in joint stiffness, pain, and general health. Food sources of carotenoids include sweet potatoes, carrots, kale, spinach, turnip greens, winter squash, collard greens, cilantro, and fresh thyme. To maximize the availability of the carotenoids in these foods, they should be eaten raw or lightly steamed. Sources of flavonoids include apples, apricots, blueberries, pears, raspberries, strawberries, black beans, cabbage, onions, parsley, pinto beans, and tomatoes.

In a 1993 study by a university in Oslo, Norway, which placed a group of fibromyalgia patients on a three-week vegetarian diet, seven out of ten fibromyalgia patients reported an increase in overall health, in the form of improved well-being and reduced pain.

A more recent double-blind, placebo-controlled trial suggests that administering pure anthocyanidins (80 milligrams daily) may be beneficial in fibromyalgia patients. Anthocyanidins are phytonutrients found in berries. Berries are the highest in anthocyanidins, powerful purple pigment compounds that act as potent antioxidants, and include vitamin C. The anthocyanidins help ease joint pain through their antioxidant activity, and they also detoxify tissues and promote better digestion. The fibromyalgia patients in the active treatment group received an anthocyanidins formula derived from cranberry, bilberry, and grape seed. The group receiving the anthocyanidins specifically reported a reduction in fatigue and improved sleep.

People whose diets are rich in fruits and vegetables live healthier lives, because these foods contain thousands of phytonutrients that interact in ways to prevent certain diseases and boost overall health. More than a hundred phytochemicals have been identified, and many have a regulating effect on the immune and endocrine system.

How Do Phytonutrients Protect Against Disease?

Phytonutrients are being studied intensively, because they have so many beneficial effects on the human body. These include:

- their antioxidant effect
- enhancing immune response
- enhancing cell-to-cell communication
- altering estrogen metabolism

- converting to vitamin A (beta-carotene is metabolized to vitamin A)
- causing cancer cells to die (apoptosis)
- repairing DNA damage caused by smoking and other toxic exposures
- detoxifying carcinogens by activating detoxification pathways within the liver

It is clear that phytonutrients play a vital part in the human body's tissue growth and repair processes and can support many more beneficial functions.

The chart below outlines the common classes of phytonutrients, the food sources in which they are found, and their specific disease-fighting powers.

In Part II, we will see which phytonutrients can be included in our diets, to help win the battle against fibromyalgia.

Phytonutrients: Where They Come From and What They Do

Phytonutrient	Source	Power
Carotenoids (more than 600) especially beta-carotene, lycopene	Red, green, yellow, and orange fruits and vegetables (especially carrots, sweet potatoes, winter squash, tomatoes, citrus, melons, cruciferous vegetables)	Antioxidants; reduce accumulation of plaque in arteries; promote cell differentiation (cancer cells are undifferentiated)
Flavonoids (more than 800) especially rutin, hesperidin, and quercetin	Most fruits and vegetables (especially citrus, onions, apples, grapes, tea)	Antioxidants that block carcinogens; suppress malignant changes; keep collagen healthy; protect eyes and nerves from inflammation and damage from diabetes; improve symptoms of allergies, asthma, and arthritis
Ellagic acid	Strawberries, grapes, raspberries, apples	Neutralize cancer-causing chemicals found in tobacco smoke, processed foods, and barbecued meats

Phytonutrient	Source	Power
Phenolic acids	Most fruits and vegetables (especially citrus, whole grains, berries, tomatoes, peppers, parsley, carrots, cruciferous vegetables, squash, yams)	Help resist cancer by inhibiting cell proliferation induced by carcinogens in target organs; inhibit platelet activity; decrease inflammation; act as antioxidants
Indoles	Cruciferous vegetables, such as broccoli, cabbage, kale	Block cancer-causing substances before they can damage cells
Isothiocyanates, *such as sulforphane*	Cruciferous vegetables	Induce protective enzymes; suppress tumor growth
Lignans	Flaxseeds, berries, whole grains	Antioxidants and insoluble fibers; block or suppress cancerous changes; anti-inflammatory; particularly protective against colon cancer and heart disease
Saponins	Garlic, onions, legumes, soybeans	Inhibit tumor promoters induced by excessively fatty diet; lower circulating levels of fats
Protease inhibitors	All plants, especially soybeans	Reduce inflammation of arthritis; anti-viral and antibacterial; suppress enzyme production in cancer cells, which may slow tumor growth
Terpenes	Oranges, lemons, grapefruit	Induce protective enzymes; interfere with action of carcinogens; prevent dental decay; anti-ulcer activity
Capsaicin	Hot peppers	Reduces pain sensation; anti-inflammatory; prevents the activation of cancer-causing chemicals
Coumarins	Soybeans, whole grains, citrus, cruciferous vegetables, cucumbers, squash, melons, parsley, flaxseeds, green tea	Anticancer activists; blood thinners
Isoflavones, *such as genistein and daidzein*	Soybeans, tofu, soy milk	Antioxidants that block carcinogens; suppress tumor formation; block estrogen from entering cells to reduce risk of breast and ovarian cancer
Organosulfurs, *such as allicin and diallyl disulfide*	Garlic, onions, leeks, chives, shallots, scallions	Block or suppress cancer-causing agents; inhibit cholesterol synthesis; boost immunity; prevent infection; help resist cancer by inhibiting nitrosamine formation and interfering with cancer-causing enzymes

Enzymes, the Keys of Life

Enzymes are another vital link in the foods that help win the battle against fibromyalgia. They support life and promote energy and vitality, and without them we can easily become fatigued and run-down. Protein carriers charged with vital energy factors, enzymes contain the power of life itself. They can be compared to a car battery, which consists of metal plates charged with electrical energy.

There are three classes of enzymes: metabolic enzymes, which run our bodies; digestive enzymes, which digest our food; and food enzymes from raw foods, which start food digestion. Our organs and tissues are run by metabolic enzymes, each organ and tissue with its own particular enzyme to do specialized work. Because good health relies on these metabolic enzymes doing an excellent job, we must be sure that nothing interferes with the body's manufacturing of them. For the body to produce these enzymes, it needs nutrients. Literally thousands of enzymes carry out various functions, and distinct enzymes run specific organs, such as the brain, liver, heart, lungs, kidneys, and so on. Even thinking involves enzyme activity. They are necessary to carry on the work of the body—repairing damage and decay and alleviating disease.

Nature's plan calls for food enzymes to help with digestion, instead of forcing the body's metabolic enzymes to carry the whole load. Food enzymes aid digestion by starting the process, leaving less work for the body's digestive enzymes. Conserving all that potential energy provides a boost in *your* overall energy.

Digestive enzymes have three main jobs: digesting protein, carbohydrate, and fat. Other enzymes do much more than help digestion and all other metabolic processes work; they literally direct the life force into our basic biochemistry. This has countless benefits, ranging from repairing our DNA and RNA to fighting disease. Enzymes are particularly effective in helping to provide more energy to the cells, because they work within the cellular structure and the cell nucleus and its energy-producing mitochondria.

Many people with fibromyalgia suffer from malnutrition and digestive problems. It has been firmly established that a central nervous system dysfunction exists with fibromyalgia and is primarily responsible for the increased pain sensitivity. Because an imbalance of the central nervous system affects the digestive system, People with fibromyalgia experience digestive problems, which eventually lead to malabsorption. Research shows that these patients suffer from a lack of the amylase enzymes early in life. These enzymes are the catalysts that break down carbohydrates. Clinical work has demonstrated that people with fibromyalgia have digestive problems with carbohydrates.

Many are also deficient in lipase enzymes, the catalysts that break down fats. Insufficient lipase enzymes can cause fatty acid and hormonal imbalances, which in turn can lead to a deficiency of protease—the enzyme that breaks down proteins. Because the protein invaders in our body are bacteria, fungal forms, and parasites—and because 70 percent of the immune system is located in the gastrointestinal tract—not surprisingly, the immune system becomes compromised.

Fortifying the body with enzyme-laden foods, such as raw (also referred to as living) foods, has proven successful in treating people with fibromyalgia. Enzymes encourage cell nutrition by feeding and strengthening the nervous system, digestive system, and endocrine (hormonal) system. Supplementing the diet with high-quality, pH-balanced digestive enzymes when eating cooked or prepared foods is also highly recommended.

Enzymes from Raw Food

Enzymes are readily found in raw foods, but their life energy can be destroyed by even moderate cooking—that is, heating food to a temperature of more than 118°F (48°C). Professor Arturo Virtanen, a biochemist and Nobel Prize winner, showed that, as digestive enzymes are released in the mouth to start the act of digestion, so too are food enzymes released when raw vegetables are chewed. These food enzymes contribute significantly to digestion, because they are not destroyed by stomach acid, as some researchers have suggested, but remain active throughout the digestive tract. Extensive tests have shown that the human body has a way of protecting enzymes that pass through the stomach, so that more than half reach the colon intact.

Some foods contain enzyme blockers (also called enzyme-inhibitors), but, as we will see in Part II, they can be defeated by food preparation strategies. Eating a raw (live) food diet helps maintain the quality and quantity of our enzyme pool and, by extension, our health and longevity. Eat fresh raw foods regularly, because they are a cocktail of essential vitamins, minerals, amino acids, antioxidants, phytonutrients, and enzymes that work together synergistically to promote energy and good health.

Antioxidants: Protectors of the Body

Antioxidants are natural compounds found in foods that help protect the body from harmful free radicals. Free radicals are atoms or groups of atoms that can cause damage to cells. In one way or another, free radicals are involved in the progression of almost every ailment, including fibromyalgia, because of the oxidative stress they cause. According to several studies, the generation of excess free radicals and/ or a deficiency in antioxidant status has been shown to play a role in fibromyalgia. Today's most exciting research implicates oxidative damage as an underlying problem in fibromyalgia, because fibromyalgia patients have measurable increases in oxidative stress.

Scientists have also observed decreased levels of red blood-cell magnesium, plasma selenium, and glutathione and alpha lipoic acid levels (all essential for antioxidants to diffuse free radicals) in people with fibromyalgia. Free radicals impair the immune system and lead to degenerative diseases including heart disease, cancer, and fibromyalgia. Oxidative stress creates more rapid aging, because of the damage it causes throughout the body. In fact, the common denominator in the process of aging and its associated diseases is oxidative damage. Antioxidants therefore play a powerful role in the prevention of disease.

There are a number of ways in which your body forms free radicals and you become oxidized: through exposure to radiation, including exposure to the sun's rays; through exposure to toxic chemicals such as those found in cigarette smoke, polluted air, eating fried and burned foods, and industrial and household chemicals; and through various metabolic processes, such as the intake of too many calories (eating more than you need), and the body's process of breaking down stored fat molecules for use as an energy source.

Diet can have a profound effect on antioxidant levels in the human body. The effect of a vegetarian diet on antioxidant levels has been the source of considerable research in recent years. Total antioxidant availability can be significantly increased by following a vegetarian diet, which is associated with increased magnesium intake and glutathione levels. One study conducted by the University of Oslo showed numerous health improvements for people with fibromyalgia. After placing fibromyalgia patients on a three-week vegetarian diet, 70 percent of the patients reported reduction of pain and improvement in overall well-being. Another study published in Scandinavia that examined the role of vegetarian, vegan, and raw (living) food diets addressed the potential role of antioxidants on fibromyalgia and arthritis patients. The results showed significant improvement in joint stiffness, pain, sleep quality, and general health. The researchers attributed the beneficial effects to the increased antioxidant levels as well as to the positive change in the intestinal microflora in the digestive tract, which helps guard against disease.

The Most Vital Antioxidants

Free radicals are normally kept in check by the action of "free-radical scavengers," which occur naturally in the body and neutralize free radicals. Certain enzymes serve this vital function. Four important enzymes neutralize free radicals: superoxide dismutase; methionine reductase; catalase; and glutathione peroxidase, and the body produces these as a matter of course. However, nutrition provides the main essential antioxidant vitamins A, C, E, and beta-carotene (the precursor of vitamin A). Beta-carotene is found in red, orange, and yellow vegetables and fruits. Vitamin C is also abundant in vegetables and fruits when eaten raw, but heat rapidly destroys it. Vitamin E is found in seed foods, including nuts and seeds (and the oils derived from them), and vegetables such as peas, broad beans, corn, and whole grains. Because frying destroys antioxidants, it is better to steam, bake, or stir-fry them.

Another antioxidant and powerful free-radical neutralizer is the hormone melatonin. Secreted by the pineal gland in the brain, melatonin is a naturally occurring hormone that helps regulate other hormones and maintain the body's circadian rhythm. The circadian rhythm is a 24-hour, internal time-keeping system that plays a critical role in determining when we fall asleep and when we wake up. It is also produced in the retina of the eye when light is low, signaling that it is time to sleep. Exposure to excessive light in the evening or too little light during the day can disrupt the body's normal melatonin cycles. Jet lag, shift work, and poor vision can disrupt melatonin cycles, as can exposure to low-frequency electromagnetic fields, which are common in household appliances. Taking melatonin supplements can help restore the body's rhythm, but they cause drowsiness, so they are best taken before bedtime. Before taking this or any supplement, you should first consult your doctor to determine if you need it and in what dosage. Certain herbs, such as ginkgo biloba, dandelion, milk thistle, and many others, have antioxidant properties, as well.

Given the unquestionable value of increasing your antioxidant levels, it is wise to make sure that your daily supplement program contains significant quantities of antioxidants, especially if you are middle-aged or older, live in a polluted city, or suffer unavoidable exposure to free radicals. The easiest way to ensure that you're giving your body an adequate supply is to take a comprehensive antioxidant supplement, in addition to consuming a full range of fresh fruits and vegetables, whole grains, nuts, and seeds.

Macronutrient Balancing: Protein, Fat, and Carbohydrates

Your body is composed entirely of molecules derived from food. Over your lifetime, you will eat 100 tons of food, which is broken down by enzymes in the digestive tract at a rate of approximately twenty-one pints (or ten liters) per day. The three main classes of foods from which we derive most of our nutrition are called *macronutrients*. They consist of proteins, fats, and carbohydrates, and we will discuss each one in more detail, because each plays an essential role in properly managing fibromyalgia.

The chart on the next page explains macronutrients in greater detail.

In addition to macronutrients are nutrients known as *micronutrients*. These are the vitamins and minerals that are absorbed through the digestive tract from our foods and from supplements.

Macronutrients: Protein, Fats, and Carbohydrates

	Protein	Fat	Carbohydrate
Food source	Meat, poultry, dairy	Oil, nuts, meat, cheese	Fruits, vegetables, grains
How your body breaks it down	Breaks down into amino acids	Breaks down into fatty acids and triglycerides	Breaks down into sugar and starch
Metabolic role	Main structural ingredient of human cells, and the enzymes that keep them running	Structural component of cell membranes, a source of insulation, and a means of energy storage	Primary source of energy for all living things, and a structural component of cell walls

Eating Right for Your Metabolism

Eating a variety of foods that contain the highest-quality nutrients in the right quantities of macronutrients helps you achieve your highest potential for health, vitality, and freedom from disease. But what are the "right" quantities of macronutrients for each individual, and how do we find them? Given that we are individually as unique in our biochemistry and metabolism as we are in our fingerprints, suffice it to say, there is no single diet that's perfect for every body. The best diet is the one that provides foods and nutrients that enable our cells to function at peak efficiency and are the most compatible with our own body chemistry.

A crucial first step in identifying the appropriate diet for you is to look at the imbalances that presently exist within your body, in terms of electrolytes and trace minerals and their ratios. Minerals, and the ratios within which they operate, as well as the accumulation of heavy metals within the body, are important bio-markers that reveal a great deal about a person's metabolic individuality, or style of functioning, and how effectively their immune system performs. Tests, including hair tissue mineral analysis, can reveal important information—such as tissue pH alkalinity, electrolyte imbalances, an underactive thyroid, and the toxicity level (for example, the presence of mercury) within the body—and

can help remove the guesswork from dietary therapy. But one of the most significant findings bears an understanding of the relationship between the oxidative system and autonomic nervous system (ANS), because this relationship provides greater insight into a one's individual metabolism. When we learn which of the two systems is the more dominant, we can recommend exactly the right kinds of foods and nutrients and the proper ratio of macronutrients for that person's system.

The rate at which cells convert food into energy, or the rate of cellular oxidation, needs to be kept in balance if the body is to function properly. Some people are fast oxidizers, meaning that their cells rapidly convert food into energy. To sustain metabolic balance, these people need foods that burn slowly, such as heavier proteins and fats. Slow oxidizers are able to maintain metabolic balance with lighter food (carbohydrates) that burns faster than protein and fat. The autonomic nervous system is the master regulator of metabolism; it plays a pivotal role in determining metabolic individuality and in influencing health and disease.

Taking a Deeper Look at the Nervous System

There are two separate branches of the autonomic nervous system. The *sympathetic* system controls bodily processes that have to do with energy utilization; it is sometimes referred to as the "fight or flight" branch. The *parasympathetic* system controls bodily activities that pertain to energy conservation; it is often thought of as the "rest and digest" branch. In most people, one branch tends to be stronger or more dominant than the other, and this creates a certain amount of biochemical or metabolic imbalance. Specific foods and nutrients have the natural capacity to strengthen the weaker side of the autonomic system. Determining whether you are "autonomic dominant" or "oxidative dominant" can explain how a food or nutrient behaves in your body—that is, whether it is alkalizing or acidifying. To select an appropriate diet and effectively balance a person's body chemistry, it is essential first to determine which system is dominant.

Evidence suggests that a diet containing the right balance of macronutrients for your particular metabolism, along with an abundance of vitamins, minerals, and essential fatty acids, is the best diet for overall health, longevity, and maintaining a healthy weight. Three general metabolic/nutritional type categories provide an effective starting point that will enable you to customize a diet that's right for you. These are protein-type, carbohydrate-type, and mixed-type, each with recommended proportions of carbs, fats, and proteins.

Protein-type:	40% protein / 30% fat / 30% carbohydrate
Carb-type:	25% protein / 15% fat / 60% carbohydrate
Mixed-type:	30% protein / 20% fat / 50% carbohydrate

The diet that works best for you is the one whose macronutrient balance most closely matches your metabolism, and it's up to you to discover the macronutrient ratio that works best for you. Once you recognize your metabolic individuality and eat according to your needs, eating becomes a pleasurable experience, rather than a complex

challenge. Identifying with certainty the kinds of meals or snacks that make you feel great and give you high levels of sustainable energy and endurance for hours at a time puts you in control of the food you eat and not the other way around. Eating becomes what it should be—easy and enjoyable. To learn more about metabolic/nutritional typing and customizing your diet, you will find detailed information on www.fodsforfybromyalgia.com and free tests to do to determine your type.

Nutrient Density

One of the best ways to assess a food's value is to determine whether it has *nutrient density*. A food's nutrient density is the amount of vitamins, minerals, essential fatty acids, and protein it has relative to its caloric content. The more nutrient-dense a food is, the more it promotes health. Following are some examples:

- Raw nuts and seeds, particularly raw almonds and fresh walnuts, and flaxseeds and flaxseed oils—these are particularly rich in essential fatty acids, vitamin E, magnesium, zinc, potassium, and fiber
- Whole grains, such as quinoa, brown rice, beans, and legumes.
- Organic produce—fruits and vegetables, particularly those that are organically grown, are high in vitamins, minerals, fiber, and phytonutrients

When we eat as Mother Nature intended us to, and we eat fresh foods that are in their most natural state, rather than being processed and devitalized, we reclaim our health and well-being.

Protein

Protein, the basic material of all living cells, is found throughout the body in muscle, bone, skin, hair, and virtually every other body part and tissue. It makes up the enzymes that power many chemical reactions and the hemoglobin that carries oxygen in your blood. Some twenty-five basic building blocks, called amino acids, are pieced together in varying combinations to make different kinds of protein. Following genetic instructions, the body strings together amino acids to make you what you are and to keep you that way.

There are eight basic essential amino acids, without which the body cannot function. Most of the remaining seventeen amino acids can be manufactured in the body when supplied with the right ingredients of protein-rich foods. Because the body doesn't store amino acids, as it does fats or carbohydrates, it needs a daily supply of them to make new protein. If a shortage of amino acids becomes chronic, which can occur if the diet is deficient in essential amino acids, the protein building process stops, and the body suffers.

Amino acids from proteins are used to make the neurotransmitters that allow your brain cells to network and communicate. Made from amino acids obtained from the protein in your food, neurotransmitters are the brain chemicals that motivate or sedate us and also help us to focus and think. Their complex interaction is what shifts your mood and changes your mind. For this reason, it's important to start the day by eating a nourishing breakfast that contains protein, because this helps to switch on the brain. If you skip breakfast, your body goes into starvation mode and starts to consume muscle. Make breakfast your most nutritious meal of the day, and notice how much more stable your energy levels become and how your ability to concentrate and focus improves.

Protein Food Sources

The best-quality protein foods, in terms of amino acid balance, are free-range organic eggs, quinoa, soybeans, beans, lentils, fish, and meat. Animal protein sources are not always the most desirable forms of protein, because they also contain a lot of undesirable fat. Also, unless the meat is organic and free range, it's likely to contain antibiotics and hormones, which the animal stores in its fat cells.

There is a concern that these can get transferred to your metabolism and cells when you eat the meat and its fat.

Meat is also acid-forming for blood pH levels, which leads to the loss of minerals, including calcium—hence the greater risk of osteoporosis among frequent meat eaters. Hormone-treated cows (particularly dairy cows) can be prone to getting infected udders, typically leading to the use of more antibiotics to treat the cows, which in turn leads to a greater residue of antibiotics remaining in the milk.

Repeated exposure to antibiotic residues in meat and dairy products over the long term is a health concern for people. Here's why: We have bacteria that live in our gut and mouth that help digest food. These friendly bacteria do not normally cause disease, because the immune system keeps them in check. If, however, the immune system is weak—generally the case with fibromyalgia or chronic fatigue syndrome—these friendly bacteria can invade tissues and cause infection. Bacteria in the body that regularly come across small amounts of antibiotics can develop ways to survive the antibiotics and become "antibiotic resistant." Should infection and illness set in, it becomes more difficult to battle these resistant bacteria with the available antibiotics.

If you decide to eat meat, limit consumption to two or three meals a week, and choose meat from animals that have been raised without the use of harmful antibiotics or hormones and from farms where they have been permitted to roam free, rather than being raised in indoor feed lots.

Some studies have shown that tryptophan levels are low in people with Fibromyalgia. Tryptophan, a chemical that contributes to overall good feelings, is the dietary raw material for manufacturing the neurotransmitter serotonin. It is needed by and stored mostly in the brain, and it can reduce both the chronic pain and the sleep difficulties associated with fibromyalgia. Evidence suggests that tryptophan might be beneficial for treating fibromyalgia, because low levels of serotonin can decrease a person's pain-tolerance threshold.

Protein-rich foods containing large quantities of neutral amino acids, found mainly in animal protein, are reported to lower brain tryptophan levels. This is because tryptophan requires the use of a transport molecule to cross the blood-brain barrier. However, in addition to tryptophan, several other amino acids—tyrosine, phenylalanine, valine, leucine, and isoleucine, for example—"compete" for this transport molecule, and their presence can inhibit the transport of tryptophan to your brain. The protein in the food you eat is made up of strands of amino acids. Eating a food high in tryptophan from meat is therefore not the best way to raise serotonin levels, and limiting such proteins by excluding animal protein from the diet has been shown to reduce pain and disease.

Complex carbohydrate foods, such as fruits, vegetables, and whole grains, are better choices. These foods contain high levels of tryptophan, without the other competing amino acids, thereby allowing the tryptophan to enter the blood, flow into the brain, and raise serotonin levels effectively. Vegetable protein sources also contain beneficial complex carbohydrates and are less acid forming. Many vegetables, especially seed foods such as beans, peas, and broccoli, contain good levels of protein and help to neutralize excess acidity. Vegetables are higher in mineral, vitamin, and fiber content and tend to be anti-inflammatory, making them a better source of protein than other foods and the most likely choice for winning the battle against fibromyalgia.

How Much Protein Do We Need?

Most Americans eat too much protein, largely as the result of a diet high in meat and dairy products. When we choose vegetables, grains, nuts, and seeds as our main protein sources, we must

ensure that we are eating generously of these foods in meals and snacks throughout the day. Choose a wide variety of protein-rich foods, to provide the body with a full complement of amino acids. Knowing whether your metabolism is a fast or slow oxidizer will also help you to determine the right ratio of proteins to include in your diet.

Fats and Oils

Fats and oils (also referred to as fatty acids) in their natural state are necessary to promote health. Essential fatty acids (EFAs) are vital components of fats and oils that cannot be produced by the body naturally, so it's essential that we get them from dietary sources. EFAs are necessary for many of the body's functions, such as a healthy nervous system and healthy skin, and they serve as natural anti-inflammatory agents.

Problems can arise as a result of eating too much of the wrong kinds of fat. The *kind* of fat and the *balance* of various fats are critical in determining how fat contributes to disease. When we do not pay attention to proper fatty acid balance, we can develop serious health problems, most of which affect the brain and the central nervous system.

Several studies have shown that people with fibromyalgia and/or chronic fatigue syndrome have essential fatty acid deficiencies and imbalances. Because essential fatty acids play an important role in forming the delicate structures that make up your brain and nervous system, they are vital to include in your daily diet. The trend toward high-carbohydrate, low-fat diets has caused many people to eat in an imbalanced way, which has affected their ratios of omega-6 to omega-3 essential fatty acids. Today, the ratio is estimated to be from 20 to 30:1, meaning that we consume twenty to thirty parts omega-6 fatty acids for every one part of omega-3 fatty acids. Years ago, our diets contained omega-6 and omega-3 fatty acids in about a one-to-one ratio (1:1), or one gram of omega-6 oils for every gram of omega-3 oils—a ratio that scientists believe is ideal for human brain function. Scientists continue to offer evidence that, when ratios of omega-6 to omega-3 fatty acids are returned to healthy balance through proper diet and nutritional supplementation, good health returns, as well.

The major problem with fats is not caused by eating too much fat so much as it is by eating too little, particularly too few essential fatty acids, such as omega-3s and omega-6s. Essential fatty acids are found in fish, nuts, seeds, oils, and vegetables.

Omega-3 Food Sources

Alpha-linolenic acid is the principal omega-3 fatty acid, which a healthy human with good nutrition will convert into eicosapentaenoic acid (EPA) and later into docosahexaenoic acid (DHA). EPA and gamma-linolenic acid (GLA) are later converted into hormone-like compounds known as eicosanoids. Eicosanoids aid in many bodily functions, including vital organ function and intracellular activity.

Omega-3s are found in foods such as flaxseed oil (which has the highest linolenic content of any food), flaxseed meal, Brazil nuts, sesame seeds, avocados, walnuts, dark green leafy vegetables (kale, spinach, purslane, mustard greens, collards), wheat germ oil, and cold-water fish, such as salmon, tuna, sardines, anchovies, and mackerel.

Omega-6 Food Sources

Linoleic acid is the primary omega-6 fatty acid. A healthy human with good nutrition will convert linoleic acid into gamma linolenic acid (GLA), which in turn is synthesized, with EPA from the omega-3 group, into eicosanoids.

Although most Americans get more than enough linoleic acid, it frequently fails to get converted to GLA due to metabolic problems caused by diets high in sugar, alcohol, or trans fats, or by smoking, pollution, stress, aging, viral infections, and other illnesses, such as diabetes. It is therefore recom-

mended that these factors be reduced or eliminated. In addition, supplementing with GLA-rich foods such as borage oil, evening primrose oil, and black currant seed oil would be beneficial.

Omega-6s are primarily found in flaxseed oil, flaxseeds, flaxseed meal, hempseeds, hempseed oil, olives, olive oil, borage oil, evening primrose oil, black currant seed oil, pumpkin seeds, pine nuts, pistachio nuts, sunflower seeds, sesame seeds, sesame oil, and chicken.

Coconut oil is also helpful in combating fibromyalgia and other immune-deficiency conditions, because it contains high levels of a medium-chain fatty acid called lauric acid (also referred to as laurate) and another called caprylic acid, both of which have been helpful in inhibiting viruses. Typical refined coconut oil contains approximately 50 percent lauric acid and 5 to 10 percent caprylic acid. These fatty acids are readily absorbed by the body and used for energy. Lauric and caprylic acid compounds have also proven to be antiviral, antibacterial, and antifungal, making coconut oil an excellent supplement for intestinal disorders, which are common in fibromyalgia. Coconut oil is stable, even during long periods of storage. Because its melting point is 75 to 76°F (24°C), coconut oil can be used in either liquid or solid form, making it ideal for cooking and baking.

Carbohydrates— Simple and Complex

Carbohydrates are probably the most important of the three main classes of foods, because they are our main source of energy. Carbohydrates come in two forms: *simple* (also called *fast-releasing* and *complex* (also known as *starch* and considered *slow-releasing*). Most sugars, sweets, refined foods, white flour, malts, and honey are fast-releasing, because they tend to produce a sudden burst of energy followed by a slump. In addition, refined foods such as sugar and flour lack the vitamins and minerals the body needs to use them properly, and so they are best avoided. When you eat slow-releasing or complex carbohydrates, such as whole grains, vegetables, beans, and lentils, or simpler carbohydrates such as fruit, the body does exactly what it is designed to do. It digests the foods and gradually releases their potential energy. What's more, all the nutrients that the body needs for digestion and metabolism are present in those whole foods. These foods also contain a less digestible type of carbohydrate called fiber, which helps keep the digestive system running smoothly.

Many people with fibromyalgia tend to have hypoglycemia—which refers to the body's inability to maintain normal levels of sugar in the blood. Sugar (or glucose) is the main source of fuel for the body, and sugar levels must remain steady, so that the brain and other organs can function normally. It is estimated that at least 75 percent of the population is hypoglycemic (a conservative figure, depending on which studies you read). Some doctors have coined the phrase "fibroglycemia" as a way of explaining that fibromyalgia patients tend to have the condition. Based on the theory that fibromyalgia is a nutritional and cellular problem that can be remedied by diet, nutrition, exercise, and stress control, this makes perfect sense.

When you eat a starchy food in its whole and unrefined state, your body breaks it down over several hours of digestion into glucose, which, as it is absorbed into the bloodstream, maintains your blood sugar, or blood glucose, level. But when you eat too much sugar or refined carbohydrates, your body overproduces insulin, which swiftly drops blood sugar to undesirably low levels. Diabetes is an extreme form of blood sugar imbalance that arises when the body fails to produce sufficient insulin, a hormone that helps carry glucose out of the blood and into cells. Some of the following problems can occur when we have low blood sugar:

- Food cravings, especially for sugary and starchy foods
- Depression
- Fatigue
- Headaches
- Anger
- Premenstrual syndrome (PMS)
- Inability to concentrate
- Dizziness
- Fainting
- Panic attacks

At one time or another, each of us has probably experienced symptoms of low blood sugar, which, if left unchecked, can develop into more serious disorders such as fibromyalgia. If we are tired or moody because we have not eaten for hours, it's a sign that our blood sugar is low. Glucose stores become depleted overnight, resulting in low blood sugar, so it is important to eat a breakfast that includes carbohydrates, protein, and healthy fats. Anyone who makes a habit of missing breakfast will experience the effects of glucose depletion, which can manifest itself in behavioral disturbances or the inability to concentrate. If we continually skip breakfast, we put added stress on our adrenal glands and pancreas, leading to reactive hypoglycemia—and this can eventually lead to diabetes. Chronic hypoglycemia is a sign that the organs that help balance blood sugar, such as the adrenal glands and the pancreas, aren't doing a good enough job and may be exhausted from overwork and too much stress. Fortunately, the symptoms of hypoglycemia can be eliminated with a nutritious diet of whole foods, frequent meals, and carefully chosen nutritional supplements.

Fiber

Fiber is a vitally important form of carbohydrate. Fiber includes cellulose, hemicellulose, pectin, and gums, and it is sometimes called bulk or roughage. There are two basic types of fiber: soluble fiber and insoluble fiber, both of which are undigested. They are not absorbed into the bloodstream but instead work to promote efficient waste from the colon and increase the bulk of feces. The bulk helps to push food along the gut, thereby reducing bowel transit time and constipation. Soluble fiber forms a gel when mixed with liquid, while insoluble fiber does not. Insoluble fiber passes through our intestines largely intact.

Sources of soluble fiber include vegetables such as carrots, fruits such as oranges and apples, barley, oat bran, dried beans and peas, nuts, and psyllium husk. Sources of insoluble fiber include vegetables such as green beans and those with dark green leaves; fruit skins; and root vegetable skins; whole-wheat products, corn bran, nuts, and seeds.

Fiber has several important health benefits. It retains water, resulting in softer and bulkier stools, which prevent constipation and hemorrhoids. A high-fiber diet also reduces the risk of colon cancer by keeping the digestive tract clean. In addition, fiber binds with certain substances that would normally result in the production of cholesterol and eliminates these substances from the body. In this way, a high-fiber diet helps lower blood cholesterol levels and reduces the risk of heart disease. Aim to eat at least 35 grams of fiber a day; 50 to 60 grams per day is even better.

Slow-releasing complex carbohydrate foods—fresh fruit, vegetables, legumes, and whole grains—provide the highest nutrient density and are an efficient form of fuel to keep your energy levels sustained for several hours. Your goal every day should be to:

- Eat six to nine servings of dark green vegetables, such as watercress, broccoli, brussels sprouts, spinach, green beans, and green peppers—either raw or lightly cooked. Eat two to four servings daily of root vegetables, such as carrots, potatoes, onions, garlic, turnips, and parsnips.
- Eat one or two servings of fresh fruit, such as apples, pears, berries, melons, or citrus fruit.
- Eat three or four servings of whole grains, such as whole-grain brown rice, millet, rye, oats, whole wheat, quinoa, or legumes.
- Avoid any form of sugar, foods with added sugar, white flour, and unrefined foods.

The Glycemic Index—Not All Carbohydrates Are Created Equal

Here's another way to look at fast-releasing and slow-releasing carbohydrates. Some carbohydrate-rich foods put more stress than others on the system that controls the body's blood sugar. Some foods cause the blood sugar level to rise rapidly, while others have almost no adverse effects on blood sugar control.

The discovery that different carbohydrates affect blood sugar differently led to the development of what is called the *glycemic index* of foods. This is the rate at which the sugars or carbohydrates in a food enter the bloodstream. When you eat packaged or highly processed foods, they quickly become absorbed by your system. This rapidly raises your blood sugar levels and causes a flood of insulin to be released from your pancreas to deal with these high levels. The high-level insulin becomes quickly depleted, and if we continue to eat such foods, we strain our pancreas, which can lead to insulin resistance and eventually to diabetes.

Foods considered to be low-glycemic are those with a GI (glycemic index) of less than 55. Foods with higher GI numbers stimulate higher blood sugar and insulin responses. Relying on low-glycemic foods can help people who are concerned about their blood sugar levels improve their health.

The next page shows a chart of glycemic index levels for some common foods.

Glycemic Index of Various Foods

Sugars	
Glucose	138
Fructose	83
Sucrose	83

Grains and Cereal Products	
Buckwheat	68
Bread (white)	100
Bread (whole grain)	60
Millet	103
Rice (brown)	54
Rice (white)	81
Pasta	67
Sweet corn	80

Breakfast Cereals	
All-Bran	74
Cornflakes	121
Muesli	96
Oatmeal	89
Shredded wheat	97

Dried Legumes	
Beans (canned)	60
Beans (kidney, dried)	43
Beans (soy)	20
Peas (black-eyed)	45
Chickpeas (garbanzos)	46
Lentils	36

Fruit	
Apples (Golden Delicious)	52
Bananas	84
Oranges	59
Orange juice	71

Dairy Products	
Ice cream	69
Milk (nonfat)	46
Milk (whole)	45
Yogurt	52

Vegetables	
Frozen peas	51
Beets	64
Carrots (raw)	16
Carrots (cooked)	36
Parsnips	96
Potato (new)	70
Potato (sweet)	48
Yam	74

Food-Combining

Food-combining involves the proper mixing or separation of foods at meals for the best digestion and for extracting as much nutrition as possible. The basic theory is that for best digestion and utilization of our food, we need to observe certain rules for the way we combine foods within a meal.

All fruits should be eaten alone (30 minutes before or 3 hours after eating) with the exception of the acid fruits—oranges, lemons, grapefruit, and cranberries—which may be eaten with protein and fats. Non-starchy and sea vegetables—asparagus, broccoli, cauliflower, kale, collards, swiss chard, spinach, cucumber, zucchini, dulse, wakame, arame, agar, kombu—can be eaten with starches (potatoes, corn, squash), grains (rice, quinoa, buckwheat), or proteins (meat, poultry, fish). The most important rule is this: Meats and starches are not eaten together at the same meal. The reason for this is that proteins require an acid digestive medium and starches an alkaline one. When combined, they interfere with each other's utilization, so that digestion takes longer and is inefficient. Eating this way generates less stress on the intestinal tract and improves your overall health and energy

Balancing Acid and Alkaline

One of the single most important indicators of health is the pH of your blood and tissues. The term pH stands for "potential of hydrogen" and is a measure of the relative acidity or alkalinity of a solution. The pH of a substance is measured on a scale from 0.00 to 14.00. The midpoint, 7.00, is neutral—neither alkaline nor acid. Water (assuming it is reasonably unpolluted) has a pH of 7.0. The lower the number, the more acidic the solution, and the higher the number, the more alkaline the solution.

All the body's fluids, with the exception of those in the stomach, depend on an alkaline environment for the metabolic process to function smoothly. Chronic over-acidity corrodes body tissue and, left unchecked, will interrupt all cellular activities and functions. An Oslo study researched the disease symptoms and diet of patients with various rheumatic disorders, including fibromyalgia. They found that 80 percent of the fibromyalgia group reported aggravation of their disease symptoms, including pain, stiffness, and joint swelling, after the intake of certain foods. Among the most offending foods were meat, wine, and coffee—all of which are highly acidic. Similar findings by investigators at the Thomas Jefferson University Hospital in Pennsylvania reported that highly acidic foods, such as red meat, pasteurized cow's milk, white flour products, sugar-containing foods, caffeine, and chocolate seem to trigger more muscle pain in people with fibromyalgia.

Because your internal systems operate in a slightly alkaline environment, the goal, then, is to create the proper alkaline balance within your body. This can be accomplished by eating the proper balance of alkaline and acidic foods. When foods are broken down by your digestive tract, a residue is left called *ash*, which can alter the body's acidity or alkalinity. Depending on its chemical composition, the ash can be acid, alkaline, or neutral.

The acidity of ash should not be confused with the intrinsic acidity of a food. Oranges and lemons, for example, are acid, due to their citric acid content. However, citric acid is completely metabolized, and the net effect of eating an orange or a lemon is to alkalize the body, hence it is classified as alkaline-forming. High-protein foods, such as meat, which make up a large portion of the standard American diet, leave acid ash. Fruits and vegetables (with a few exceptions) leave alkaline ash.

By reducing the amount of high-protein, acid ash-producing foods in your diet, your internal environmental conditions become right for optimum health. Roughly 80 percent of our diets should come from alkaline-forming foods, and 20 percent from acid-forming foods. Let's take a look at the basic four food groups—the cornerstones of most diets—to see how they stack up, in terms of their pH value.

Food Group	pH
Meats, Poultry, Fish	*Strongly Acidic*
Dairy Products, Eggs	*Acidic*
Cereals, Grains	*Acidic*
Fruits, Vegetables	*Alkaline*

When we look at the USDA's new and revised Food Guide Pyramid, we can see that the diet contains 66 percent acid-ash foods and only 33 percent alkaline-ash foods. (The longstanding original Food Guide Pyramid was even more lopsided, containing only 25 percent alkaline-ash foods.) By switching these ratios around and making fruits and especially green vegetables 75 to 80 percent of your diet, you will see immediate improvement in your health. Your energy will increase, many chronic health conditions will improve or vanish, you'll enjoy new mental clarity and powers of concentration, you'll build strength and stamina, and you'll lose excess body fat, while increasing muscle mass. Your entire body will function more efficiently, achy joints and tired muscles will disappear, and you will regain the store of energy and wellness you thought was lost completely.

Beneficial Bacteria and Probiotics

Bacterial overgrowth and yeast infections are thought to be two of the triggers that cause fibromyalgia and chronic fatigue syndrome. As the standard American diet becomes increasingly dependent on processed foods, sugars, and refined grains and our environment filled with chemicals and pollution, the result, for many of us, has been a substantial increase in harmful bacteria in our intestinal tract.

When there is an overgrowth of bacteria, yeast, fungus, or parasites inside the GI tract, the intestinal lining becomes damaged and weakened.

This permits undigested food particles, disease-causing bacteria, and potentially toxic molecules to pass directly through the weakened cell membranes and into the rest of the body, where they quickly spread. Toxins pass through the intestinal walls into the bloodstream and are carried to the liver, which becomes overworked in an effort to detoxify this increased load of toxins.

To make matters worse, the toxins circulating in our bloodstream activate antibodies and cause irritation and inflammation throughout other parts of the body, triggering a host of other distressing symptoms. This chain effect causes oxidative damage, which speeds up the aging process. Eventually, it can lead to something commonly called *leaky gut syndrome*. Symptoms associated with leaky gut syndrome include abdominal pain, chronic joint and muscle pain, gas, indigestion, brain fog, confusion, mood swings, nervousness, skin rashes, extreme fatigue, bloating, constipation, shortness of breath, diarrhea, aggression, and poor memory.

Following is a partial list of symptoms that can be triggered by an imbalance of bacteria in the GI tract:

- Fibromyalgia and chronic fatigue syndrome
- Gas, bloating, and indigestion
- Irritable bowel syndrome
- Diarrhea and constipation
- Skin problems, such as acne, eczema, and psoriasis
- Bad breath and body odor
- Candida yeast infections
- Delayed development in children
- Frequent colds and flu

Restoring Gastrointestinal Tract Health

It is critical to understand the relationship between the bacteria living in our gastrointestinal tract and its effect on our health, because the kind of bacteria your body contains in the largest numbers determines how healthy you are. A total of 100 trillion bacteria live in your GI tract—more than the number of living cells in your body. Some of these bacteria are known as *friendly* or *good* bacteria, while some are *harmful* or *bad*. Friendly bacteria keep the immune system strong and the digestive system functioning smoothly. The wrong or harmful variety of bacteria set the stage for disease.

Ideally, beneficial bacteria should make up about 85 percent of the intestinal tract's population, and harmful bacteria about 15 percent. Most Americans, however, have the inverse ratio of 15 percent good bacteria to 85 percent bad. This ratio can seriously compromise the immune and digestive systems, leading to a number of chronic conditions and disorders like fibromyalgia. Many people with fibromyalgia have additional gastrointestinal problems from the many drugs they are often prescribed. These drugs alter the levels of beneficial bacteria in the gut. For this reason, a person who has fibromyalgia should take probiotics, including the lactobacillus group of beneficial bacteria, to restore gastrointestinal function.

Lactobacillus acidophilus and bifidobacterium are the two predominant beneficial bacteria in our intestinal tract, and we need both for a healthy GI tract. These friendly bacteria are called *intestinal flora*, *probiotics*, or *eubiotics*—the last two terms meaning "healthful to life." We use the term probiotics to refer to supplemental use of these bacteria in powder or capsule form. Lactobacillus acidophilus is the bacteria most people are familiar with; however, bifidobacterium appears to be an equally important beneficial bacteria in the GI tract. Lactobacillus is particularly helpful in treating *candida albicans*, a fungus that causes thrush, yeast infections, and infections in the nails and eyes. It is thought that candida albicans yeast overgrowth is prevalent in many Fibromyalgia patients.

Friendly intestinal flora in our GI tract are also responsible for manufacturing many vitamins, including the B-complex vitamins. The B-complex vitamins are our stress-fighting vitamins, and we can only make them by eating the right foods. It's been said that our gut is our second brain, and when we fully appreciate that 70 percent of our immune system is located there, it's no wonder! We want to keep our GI tract in good order and our friendly flora in abundant supply, and the way we do this is through nutrition and diet. We can also supplement with probiotics—a necessary move when we tend to take numerous doses of antibiotics over the course of our lives. One dose of antibiotics will kill not only the harmful bacteria but *all* the bacteria living in our GI tract, including the friendly sort. It can take us up to one year to restore the friendly bacteria in our gut, unless we eat foods that contain it.

Foods That Enhance GI Flora

Most cultured and fermented foods commonly increase bacterial content, making them a rich source of friendly flora. Many cultures around the world have long recognized the benefits of fermented foods. While some indigenous peoples may not have known the science behind their use, they quickly noticed of their healthful benefits. For example, sauerkraut, a traditional European food, has a long history of use by people with ulcers and digestive problems. Asian cultures traditionally use pickles and fermented foods, such as kimchee, as condiments. Following is a list of foods containing either lactobacillus acidophilus or bifidobacterium, or both:

- Yogurt
- Sauerkraut
- Cottage cheese
- Tofu
- Miso
- Natto
- Tamari
- Shoyu
- Tempeh
- Kimchee

Chinese green tea and ginseng also increase friendly flora. Green tea contains polyphenols, which are believed to be friendly-flora enhancing, while ginseng extract has likewise been found to increase beneficial flora.

Holistic Nutrition—Creating Synergy

Now that we've looked at many of the components of nutrition, it's easier to see how they work individually and in concert. When we approach nutrition by first understanding the basic principles and the way in which each of the various components functions and then looking at nutrition holistically, we can see how synergy is created. The whole *is* greater than the sum of its parts.

Synergy within the body is created when all systems work cooperatively to provide optimum health. When you fail to provide the necessary nutritional components, synergy breaks down, leading to ill health and disease.

The subjects of food and nutrition often generate confusion, and this stems in part from the large amount of conflicting information we receive via the media. We walk through the supermarket as if it were a minefield, with our list of foods to avoid, such as fats, cholesterol, and whatever other food the media has deemed dangerous. We can clear away the confusion when we understand and practice the basic principles of healthy eating. Adopting these, we will find that everything falls into place and becomes intuitive. You will find yourself enjoying the same foods today that your great-grandparents enjoyed decades ago, the same foods that will form the nutritional centerpieces for your great-grandchildren in the decades to follow.

Summary

- We are each unique in our personal biochemistry; therefore, there is no single diet that's suitable for everyone. Through direct monitoring and control of your own nutrition, you will discover your own balance.

- Eat at least eight to ten servings of colorful fruits and vegetables every day. Eat food in as raw and unprocessed a form as possible. Avoid synthetic chemicals.
- There is no substitute for whole foods, which contain hundreds of health-promoting substances, such as phytonutrients. These play a vital part in the human body's tissue growth and repair processes and may potentially support a number of other beneficial functions.
- Try eating a mostly vegetarian or vegan diet, with close to 70 percent of your food consisting of fruits, vegetables, seed sprouts, nuts, and seeds. If you eat meat, avoid meat from animals raised in feed-lots with hormones and antibiotics, and try to choose fish or organic, free-range game instead. Eat these foods no more than three times per week and always with vegetables.
- Enzymes contain the power of life itself. They are readily found in raw (living) foods, but their life-energy can be destroyed by even moderate cooking. Therefore, eat generous amounts of raw salads every day.
- Antioxidants are natural compounds found in foods that help protect the body from harmful free radicals, which lead to aging and chronic disease. Fruits and vegetables are rich sources of antioxidants.
- When you switch from an acid to an alkaline pH, it will make all the difference to your health. An alkaline system helps keep your GI tract free from harmful bacteria, yeast, and parasites. Fruits and vegetables are the most alkalizing foods available. Remember, 70 percent of your immune system is located in your gut.

CHAPTER 5

YOUR LIFESTYLE GUIDE: SHOPPING LISTS AND EATING TIPS

This chapter will outline a plan to help you take charge of your health and feel good on every level. As with every aspect of maintaining your well-being, healthy cooking involves certain principles, which we'll discuss, along with some useful techniques. Adopting healthy cooking habits is one of the most important things we can do. If you have fibromyalgia—or any other health condition—chances are that your kitchen will need a comprehensive make-over, from the foods in your pantry to the utensils you typically use. Your aim is to set up the kitchen so that it matches your new health-generating lifestyle. You want to increase the amount of nutrients and decrease the amount of toxic substances you ingest. It may cost a bit more to eat foods that are organically grown and therefore more beneficial to our health, but you are worth it! You can spend money on the best foods and fully enjoy them, or you can spend it on medications and medical bills. Your health is priceless, so the choice is obvious.

The Healthy Pantry

Nutritious cooking begins with stocking the pantry and refrigerator with healthy ingredients. The contents of the pantry may vary with the seasons, but the need to keep healthy ingredients on hand for preparing healthy meals never changes. The first step, before filling the pantry with healthy foods and ingredients, is to toss out any items that are detrimental to building optimal health. Products containing hydrogenated vegetable oil, vegetable shortening, or partially hydrogenated vegetable oils are first to go—check for them in margarine, cookies, crackers, cereals, frozen foods, breads, pastries, muffins, donuts, snack foods, salad dressings, mayonnaise, potato chips, candy bars, and other packaged foods.

The process of hydrogenation or partial hydrogenation turns liquid vegetable oils into solid vegetable shortenings. Hydrogenation converts the naturally occurring "cis" form of fat molecules into a "trans" form. In nature most unsaturated fatty acids are cis fatty acids, which means that the hydrogen atoms are on the same side of the double carbon bond. In "trans" fatty acids, the two hydrogen atoms are on opposite sides of the double bond. Trans double bonds can occur in nature as the result of fermentation in grazing animals. People eat them in small amounts in the form of meat and dairy products. However, more trans double bonds are formed during the hydrogenation and refining process of liquid vegetable oils.

Trans double bonds can be formed in monounsaturated and polyunsaturated fatty acids, and fats containing trans unsaturated fatty acids are called trans fats. Our body does not recognize this new form of fat molecule, because it is foreign to our cells. Trans fatty acids block normal biochemistry and inhibit enzymes involved in the synthesis of cholesterol and fatty acids. Consuming too many trans fats has been linked to cancer in animals and humans. Moreover, they are associated with hardening of the arteries (atherosclerosis), heart disease, and all inflammatory illnesses—including arthritis, eczema, irritable bowel syndrome, and fibromyalgia. In addition, trans fatty acids affect our body's electrical circuitry, which is responsible for all body functions, from the way our minds work to controlling heartbeat, cell division, muscle coordination, and energy levels. It's best to avoid them at all costs.

While you are cleaning out your pantry, discard the following foods, because they are devitalized and devoid of nutrients: highly processed foods, including white flour products and enriched products, foods with high sugar content, foods filled with preservatives and colorings, foods with a long shelf life, and foods past their expiration dates. Once this is done, congratulate yourself. You've taken an important step on your road to recovery and optimum health. These "foods" are filled with anti-nutrients and are loaded with calories instead of nutrients.

They have compromised your health status for too long; it's time to change and upgrade the foods we put into our bodies and reap the rewards of good health and increased vitality.

Reading Food Labels– A Wise Habit to Adopt

A food's label and overall packaging are designed to sell products. Packaging labels are therefore not a guarantee that the contents are nutritious but rather a message from the manufacturer about how healthful it hopes you will find the product.

The ingredient list on food labels is probably the most important information on the package because it discloses what's actually in the product. Armed with this information, you can learn about each ingredient and determine for yourself just how healthy it—and the overall product—is.

Finding—and comprehending—the ingredients on a label can be a challenge. Sometimes they are hidden under packaging material or appear in print that's barely legible. But it is important to get into the habit of looking for the label and reading it, to assess the product's ingredients. If a product does not have a label, it's best not to buy it. The absence of a label could mean that the product is old and out of date or that it contains ingredients we'd rather not put into our bodies. By law, all packaged goods must contain a label.

Ingredients are listed on the label in order of weight—the ingredient that weighs the most is listed first, and the ingredient that weighs the least is listed last. A general rule of thumb: If the label carries a long list of ingredients, there are probably a bunch of chemical additives in the product, and you're risking your health by eating it. The converse is not necessarily true: If the list of ingredients is short, the item may or may not have harmful additives, so read the ingredients carefully before you decide to purchase it.

Often, the package includes statements such as "Natural Fruit Flavors, with Real Fruit Juice," "All Natural Ingredients," or "No Preservatives Added." The word *natural*, however, does not always mean safe or healthy, because many products and ingredients that are natural—mushrooms, for example—can also be deadly. Because a product's ingredients are listed in order of decreasing weight, the designation "natural" may only apply to the first ingredient or primary ingredients—not all of them. The claim that a product is natural is often a complete misrepresentation and sometimes nothing more than a trade name (for example, "100% Natural Granola"). Slapping "natural" on a product does not mean it is free of harmful additives and chemicals. It is simply the manufacturer's device to persuade you to buy a product you believe is genuinely natural and therefore good for you. But many additives can masquerade as real food, when in fact they have been made in a food laboratory and are far from healthy.

As recently as December 2005, the FDA made the following statement with regard to its policy on the use of the word "natural" on food labels: "… [T]here are many facets of this issue that the agency will have to carefully consider if it undertakes a rulemaking to define the term natural. Because of resource limitations and other agency priorities, FDA is not undertaking rulemaking to establish a definition for 'natural' at this time."

Food Additives to Avoid

The average American consumes almost 150 pounds of additives per year, and almost 90 percent of that amount is sugar in one form or another. In 1990, more than 30 billion pounds of added sweeteners were consumed by the American public. Today, more than 14,000 manmade chemicals are added to our food supply. Additives have played an enormous role in the increase of both the junk food and fast food markets, through which a great many of those 150 pounds of additives are consumed.

Food additives are not natural nutrition for humans or their pets. Children suffer the most from food additives, because they are exposed to food chemicals from infancy and even before birth if the mother's diet is less than adequate. This type of exposure has a damaging effect on the growth and development of human life, with disastrous genetic ramifications for future generations. Human bodies were not meant to be exposed to the range of chemicals and food additives that we confront today.

Studies have shown that fibromyalgia patients have definite and adverse reactions to chemicals added to food. In a series of case studies published in the *Annals of Pharmacotherapy*, researchers from the University of Florida concluded that eliminating monosodium glutamate (MSG) and aspartame led to marked improvement in certain Fibromyalgia patients. Only four patient cases were described in the study, but the results were significant in that there was almost a complete resolution of symptoms within months. When these same patients were re-challenged with the offending substances, there was clear exacerbation of fibromyalgia symptoms. The evidence makes plain that eliminating MSG and aspartame (a low-cost and non-invasive method of treatment), is helpful in reducing fibromyalgia symptoms.

It is essential to recognize—and then avoid—the types of chemicals and food additives that are plentiful in today's marketplace. Following is a list of several that are engulfing our modern food supply.

Aspartame

This sugar substitute is sold commercially as Equal and NutraSweet. Aspartame has been linked to a number of health problems and should not be consumed. It consists of the amino acids aspartic acid and phenylalanine, which can lead to phenylketonuria (PKU), a condition that can cause problems with brain development. More than ninety documented symptoms have been associated with the consumption of aspartame, including altered brain function and behavioral changes. Many people report dizziness, headaches, epileptic-like seizures, and hormonal problems after ingesting aspartame. One out of 20,000 babies is born without the ability to metabolize phenylalanine, resulting in mental retardation. Do not take aspartame if you are pregnant, suffer from PKU, or have experienced side effects from taking it.

Acesulfame K

Known commercially as Sunette or Sweet One, acesulfame is a sugar substitute sold in packet or tablet form, in chewing gum, dry mixes for beverages, instant coffee and tea, gelatin deserts, puddings, and nondairy creamers. Studies have shown that this additive causes cancer in animals and may cause low blood sugar attacks.

Artificial Colorings

The majority of artificial colorings used in food are synthetic dyes. Food coloring is used to add color lost during processing, to make food look more attractive, and to make food look fresher and more natural. Various food colorings can be mixed together, and some processed goods contain more than five different added colors. These dyes are prevalent in candies and desserts that are marketed to children. Based on body weight, children often consume far more food coloring in the space of a day than is recommended, and they ingest significantly more food coloring than adults. It has been suspected for decades that artificial colorings are toxic or carcinogenic, and many have already been banned. Any food containing artificial coloring should make you question its nutritional value and should be avoided. Healthy foods with natural ingredients provide all the color you need.

Monosodium Glutamate (MSG)

MSG is found in many Asian-style cuisines but can also be found in processed and canned foods. It's used in certain seasonings to enhance or add flavor. MSG and MSG-like food additives (such as aspartame) belong to a class of compounds known as excitotoxins. Simply put, excitotoxins excite brain cells until they die. In other words, each serving of MSG has the potential to cause a little bit of brain damage, which becomes cumulative and could eventually lead to neurological diseases, such as Alzheimers and Parkinsons disease.

Many people are highly sensitive to MSG and may not know it's in their food, because it is often disguised as "hydrolyzed vegetable protein" or "HVP." MSG can cause a host of symptoms, including extreme thirst and dehydration, headaches, tightness in the chest, and a burning sensation in the forearms and back of the neck.

Caffeine

Caffeine is found naturally in coffee, tea, mate leaves, guarana root, and kola nuts. It also gets added to many soft drinks, particularly cola drinks. For any food in which it is naturally found, such as coffee, tea, or cocoa, caffeine does not need to be listed on the label. The decaffeination of coffee is a process that uses chemical solvents, such as formaldehyde. The caffeine extracted from decaffeinated coffee often goes on to be used in other food products.

Caffeine is a stimulant, affecting the heart, central nervous system, and respiratory system. Caffeine also promotes stomach-acid secretion (possibly increasing the symptoms of peptic ulcers), temporarily raises blood pressure, and dilates some blood vessels, while constricting others. Regular excessive intake leads to symptoms ranging from nervousness to insomnia.

Experiments on lab animals have linked caffeine to birth defects, such as cleft palates, missing fingers and toes, and skull malformations. A major concern is that caffeine can pass the placental barrier and affect the growing fetus; therefore, it is not recommended during pregnancy. Nor is it recommended for nursing mothers, because it enters a mother's

Food Additives and Alternatives

Additives to Avoid

Artificial colors	Artificial flavorings
Sodium nitrate	Olestra
Potassium Nitrite	TBHQ
BHT (butylated hydroxytoluene)	Propyl gallate
Saccharin	EDTA
Sulfites (especially sodium bisulfite)	Hydrogenated vegetable oils
Sulfur dioxide	Trans fats
BVO (brominated vegetable oil)	Aspartame
BHA (butylated hydroxyanisole)	Caffeine
MSG (monosodium glutamate)	Gums (guar gums, gum bases)
Sugars (sucrose, dextrose)	Propylene glycol
High-fructose corn syrup	Xylitol
Benzoic acid	Aluminum salts

Safer Alternatives

Vitamin A, C, and E	Glycerin—mono- and diglycerides
Beta-carotene or Carotene	Gelatin
Annatto	Pectin
Acids—citric, ascorbic, lastic	Lecithin
Minerals—iron, zinc, and others	Vanillin

milk. A diuretic, caffeine puts added stress on the adrenal glands and urinary system and has been shown to leach calcium from the bones.

In general, caffeine should be considered a potentially addictive drug that should not be consumed every day but taken intermittently and with caution. Experts agree that moderation and common sense are the keys here. What is a "normal" or safe amount of caffeine depends on an individual's sensitivity, which can be affected by frequency and amount of intake, body weight, age, and a person's overall health. People with health problems should consult their physician regarding their use of caffeine.

Nitrates and Nitrites (Sodium Nitrate, Potassium Nitrite [Saltpeter])

Nitrates and nitrites have been used for decades to cure ham, bacon, sausage, hot dogs, corned beef, lunch meats, and fish products. These substances convert to compounds called secondary amines, which form nitrosamines, extremely powerful cancer-causing chemicals. The chemical reaction occurs most readily at high frying temperatures. Nitrosamines have been shown to be potent carcinogens in animals, producing increased amounts of cancer in the liver, lungs, and pancreas, and they have long been suspected of causing stomach cancer in humans. Avoid all foods, especially bacon and cured meats, that contain these substances.

Healthy Eating and Shopping Pointers

1. Do most of your shopping in the outside aisles of your grocery store or supermarket. Fresh foods, such as fruits and vegetables, fresh meat, fish, and poultry, and dairy products, are typically located around the perimeter of the store. Most of the inner isles are filled with processed foods in boxes, cans, or plastic containers. These processed foods are typically calorie-dense, rather than nutrient-dense, and are filled with anti-nutrients such as chemicals, preservatives, and trans fats. These foods are also higher in sodium, sugar, and MSG, and should be avoided altogether.

2. Shop with a list. When you shop with a list tailored to your specific needs, you shop with more intention. Organize your shopping list according to the store sections you plan to visit (produce, meat, dairy, and so on). Think of them as departments of the supermarket, much like separate stores at the mall; this way, you won't spend precious time "browsing" unnecessary sections. Your shopping will be more organized, and you'll be finished more quickly, too.

3. Shop with a full stomach. When you walk through the supermarket hungry, you are susceptible to buying things that you wouldn't ordinarily purchase or that are calorie dense. If you must go shopping on an empty stomach, bring along a piece of fruit or some raw nuts, so you won't be tempted to buy unnecessary items or junk foods.

4. If you must buy pre-packaged food, always read the label. Compare similar items, and choose the one with the best-quality fat content. This would include pure-pressed extra-virgin olive oil and organic butter from grass-fed animals. "Pure-pressed" (or from the first pressing) refers to how the oil was produced and affirms that it is an unrefined, natural product that has undergone very little processing. Avoid buying anything containing MSG or any ingredients whose names you cannot pronounce or have never heard of. If an ingredient is unpronounceable or unfamiliar, there's a high likelihood that it's a chemical manufactured in a lab and is detrimental to your health and well-being.

5. Buy and eat local fresh foods in season. In other words, consume foods that are grown in your agricultural area during the season in which they are grown. Some foods, such as root vegetables, grains, nuts, and seeds, store better than others, and these can be consumed in the off-season, when most foods in many areas are not available in their fresh state. Local foods have the highest levels of nutrients and enzyme activity. They often cost less than what gets shipped in from other states (or countries), taste better than packaged and frozen foods, and have a lower risk of carrying pathogens such as E. coli. Food fresh from local farms and purveyors is simply the healthiest available.

6. Seek out and purchase organically grown foods whenever possible. Organic foods are grown without chemical fertilizers and pesticides and are therefore less toxic to your body. In addition, your efforts will support the organic food industry and help raise awareness of healthier food. Studies confirm that organically grown fruits and vegetables contain higher levels of cancer-fighting antioxidants than conventionally produced foods. Plus, mineral levels in organically grown foods have been found to be twice as high on average as commercially grown produce. Animals raised on organic farms are not fed dangerous hormones and antibiotics, which means there's no added risk that they'll be passed on to us through the food we eat.

7. Shop at local farmer's markets or co-ops, where you can learn precisely how the food was grown. The food sold at these markets tends to be fresher, less expensive, and less chemically treated than that available in supermarkets. Your patronage helps support small or family farms.

8. Buy fresh produce a few days before it ripens. There's no point in buying fresh vegetables and fruits if they turn brown and mushy a day or two after you bring them home. Unless you plan to eat it within a day or two, buy fruits and vegetables that are still firm to the touch, check expiration dates on bagged produce, and stay away from green potatoes or onions that have started to sprout. If you can't find produce in the state of ripeness you want, ask to speak to the produce manager, to see if there's more in the back waiting to be put on the shelves.

9. Avoid foods and drinks made with high-fructose corn syrup (HFCS). High-fructose corn syrup is an unhealthy form of sweetener, in the same way that trans fats are an unhealthy form of fat. High-fructose corn syrup is a calorie-dense, nutritionally empty sweetener made from corn that spikes insulin levels more rapidly than sugar. Some experts claim that high-fructose corn syrup is the main cause of America's obesity problem, and that, if everyone stopped eating it, we could dramatically reduce our national death and illness rates.

   Health experts claim that the body processes the fructose in HFCS differently from old-fashioned cane or beet sugar—a difference that alters the way metabolic-regulating hormones function. HFCS is a staple ingredient in a staggering number of foods and drinks, including such seemingly healthy foods as fruit juice, salad dressing, prepared spaghetti sauce, ketchup, and bread. Read labels, and if you see high-fructose corn syrup on the ingredient list, it would be wise to pass on that particular product.

10. Minimize the use of sugar, particularly sucrose or white sugar. In its place, try natural sweeteners, such as date sugar, rice or malt syrup, or maple syrup (preferably in that order).

Many people have taken to using agave, which is derived from the blue agave plant in Mexico. Although agave is touted in health food stores and on the Internet as safe, natural, and low-glycemic, according to Russ Bianchi, CEO of a global food formulation firm called Adept Solutions, it is "a non-GRAS (not generally recognized as safe) label for highly refined fructose, which is metabolized in your body like high-fructose corn syrup." Bianchi adds that agave has twice the intensity and sweetness of high-fructose corn syrup, and several countries have passed laws either banning it or reviewing its safety. Best to err on the side of safety and satisfy your sweet tooth by reaching for fresh fruit once or twice a day.

Honey is another sweetener that requires some clarification. While it may be naturally processed by bees, it still delivers a large dose of fructose and sucrose. When eaten as a "natural" substitute for sugar, it presents the same problems associated with sucrose: increased insulin levels, lowered immune system function, and damage to the vascular system, which can lead to heart disease, adult onset diabetes, and other health issues. Although honey contains some health-promoting compounds, such as antioxidants, and can enhance calcium absorption, it is best used in moderation and should not be thought of as a healthy replacement for sucrose.

11. Avoid red meats—beef, pork, and lamb. Raising livestock on a vast scale is destructive to the natural environment, and these animals are usually pumped full of chemicals and hormones, which make them unhealthy to eat. Whenever possible, buy meats from range-fed animals, free of antibiotics and hormones. Do not consume lunch meats or other nitrate- or nitrite-cured meats. These have been known to cause cancer and other immune- and digestive-related disorders.

12. Increase your intake of high-fiber foods, particularly vegetables, fruits, and whole grains. We need at least 30 grams of fiber per day, but as much as 50 to 60 grams per day is recommended. Americans eat an average of just 12 grams of fiber a day, which makes it hardly surprising that we have high levels of digestive disorders. We now know low-fiber diets lead to diverticulosis, appendicitis, colon polyps, colon cancer, hemorrhoids, and varicose veins. Diets high in soluble fiber are helpful for people with irritable bowel syndrome, Crohns disease, peptic ulcers, and hiatal hernias. Dietary fiber also helps prevent obesity by slowing down the rate of digestion and keeping blood sugar and insulin levels stable. Fiber has been shown to normalize serum cholesterol levels and reduce the risk of heart disease, high blood pressure, and certain types of cancer.

The foods that are the richest sources of fiber are whole grains (brown rice, whole wheat, bulgur, millet, buckwheat, rye, barley, spelt, oats), legumes (all beans except green beans), vegetables, and fruits.

13. Choose fresh foods whenever possible, opting for frozen food as a second choice. Some canned foods, such as tuna, salmon, and sardines, are okay to have on hand, but be sure they are packed in spring water, not oil. Canned tomato sauces and crushed or stewed tomatoes are another exception. Studies have shown that these actually have higher amounts of the antioxidant lycopene than fresh tomatoes, because they've become concentrated. Read the label on the can, to be sure it doesn't contain high-fructose corn syrup, added sodium, or MSG.

Never use foods from containers with these spoilage warning signs: bulging, leaking, or badly dented cans (especially along the top, side, and bottom seams); loose or bulging lids on jars; or foods with a foul odor. When storing canned food, store it in a cool, clean, dry place, try not to keep canned foods for longer than one year, and definitely use canned meats and seafood within twelve months of the purchase date (foods stored longer than a year may deteriorate in color, flavor, and nutritive value).

14. When you have to buy non-organic fruits and vegetables, check the labels on fresh and frozen produce and try to avoid foods grown in Mexico, Central America, or South America. Produce from these countries tends to be grown using chemicals that have been banned in the United States. When buying waxed produce, such as apples, cucumbers, and eggplants, peel them before cooking or eating, because pesticides are sealed in with the wax. Wash all produce thoroughly or soak it a solution made of water and a small amount of hydrogen peroxide.

15. Choose dairy products carefully. Whenever possible, buy organic milk, cheese, yogurt, butter, and ice cream. These are widely available in many health food stores and supermarkets. You may also want to consider buying *raw* milk and cheese products—these have not been pasteurized or homogenized and still have all their enzymes intact. Some states only sell raw dairy products for pet consumption or on certified farms. Search online for local organic dairy farms, to find the one closest to you.

Goat milk is another healthy alternative, especially for people who are lactose intolerant. If you like yogurt, buy it plain and flavor it at home with fruit. Flavored yogurts have plenty of sugar, which destroys any health benefits offered by the yogurt. Look for brands that contain probiotics, such as acidophilus and bifidus bacteria, to promote a healthy GI tract and immune system.

Equipping a Healthy Kitchen

One way to ensure that you create wholesome cooked food, complete with all its nutrients, is to carefully select your cookware and utensils. A whole world of useful gadgets and small appliances designed to help us eat more healthfully are available. Although these items are not essential to eating well, they can make the process easier and more fun. Using high-quality equipment helps us optimize a food's health-giving properties. It may require a small investment, but in terms of durability and results, good equipment is well worth the initial cost. To make your kitchen an enjoyable, easy place to work, make sure your tools and ingredients are accessible and your work surfaces are kept clean.

Cookware

Some of the best cookware available is made from ceramic, glass, or lead-free earthenware, because they are non-reactive. The enzymes in food, raw or cooked, are chemically active and can react with the metallic ions in metal cookware, affecting food taste and making it toxic. If you choose to cook with metal, use high-density cast iron (without a graphite coating), heavy-gauge stainless, surgical steel, or good-quality, enamel-lined cookware. Avoid aluminum cookware and "non-stick" surfaces. Teflon coatings and non-stick finishes on cookware have been known to flake off into food, and these chemicals enter your body as toxins. Foods cooked or stored in aluminum produce a substance that neutralizes the digestive juices, leading to acidosis and ulcers. Aluminum itself can leach from the cookware into food and be absorbed by the body, where it accumulates in the brain and nervous system tissues.

Aluminum is also found in unfiltered tap water, baking soda, antiperspirants, and even table salt. It is dangerous and can be fatal if consumed in excessive amounts, particularly in children and the elderly, where the blood-brain barrier is more delicate. Excessive amounts of aluminum deposits have also been implicated in Alzheimers disease.

- When cooking with metal cookware, remove food immediately after cooking so it doesn't retain a metallic taste.
- The best pots have thick bottoms that prevent burning over high heat and help distribute heat more evenly.
- Do not add acidic foods, such as lemon, tomatoes, pineapple, or vinegar, to cast iron—it will create a strong metallic taste and turn the food a dark color.

The Dangers of Microwave Cooking

Convenient as it is, microwave-oven use is best avoided. Research suggests that food prepared in a microwave shows a marked acceleration of structural degradation, which leads to a decrease in food value of 60 to 90 percent. In short, microwave cooking distorts foods' molecular structure and destroys much of its nutrient content. They are known to cause many other problems with the immune system over a period of time. In a 1989 article noted in the respected British medical journal *Lancet* on the health effects of microwave ovens, Dr. Lita Lee states that every microwave oven leaks electromagnetic radiation, harms food, and converts substances cooked in it to dangerous organ-toxic and carcinogenic products. According to Dr. Lee, consumers of microwaved foods display changes in their blood chemistries and the rates at which they develop certain diseases. Findings also showed:

- Lymphatic disorders, leading to a decreased ability to prevent certain types of cancers.
- An increased rate of cancer cell formation in the blood.

- Higher rates of digestive disorders and a gradual breakdown of the systems of elimination.

Some of the more common signs and symptoms associated with the use of microwave radiation, according to Robert O. Becker in his book *The Body Electric*, include headache, dizziness, eye pain, sleeplessness, irritability, anxiety, stomach pain, nervous tension, inability to concentrate, hair loss, and an increased incidence of appendicitis, cataracts, reproductive problems, and cancer.

The microwave's chief appeal is that it heats food quickly. This accelerated heating can lead to uneven and non-calculable heat distribution in the food, resulting in so-called "cold spots" and "hot spots." Germs are often not sufficiently inactivated and eliminated, which, for example, could cause salmonella poisoning, if chicken has not been properly heated to kill all the bacteria.

The Right Tools

The following are some tools and appliances that you will find indispensable in running your healthy kitchen.

Knives Knives are essential for cleaning, trimming, cutting, and chopping. There are three styles of knives that you will use the most: a serrated knife for bread and vegetables, a large chopping knife, and tempered (or case-hardened) steel knives for carving meat and filleting fish. Tempering is the process of heating a steel blade to high temperatures, usually a number of times, to harden it. Look for high-quality knives with a lifetime guarantee. Before purchasing a knife, try it out by holding it in the store and noticing how it feels in your hand. It should feel natural—like an extension of your hand. Care for your knives by sharpening them often, drying them after each use, and storing them in a way that protects the blades from damage.

Cutting Boards You need at least two cutting boards—one for raw proteins, such as poultry and fish, and another for vegetables, fruits, and cooked proteins. This helps avoid cross-contamination when cooking. Wood or bamboo cutting boards are more likely to harbor pathogenic bacteria than plastic ones. Treat these with oil periodically and avoid placing them in the dishwasher. Plastic cutting boards, however, can safely be cleaned in the dishwasher.

Kitchen Scissors Sturdy kitchen scissors come in handy for a variety of tasks, from snipping herbs to cutting up whole chickens.

Food Processor A food processor makes quick work of chopping and grating, which is great when you are short on time but still want to eat healthy, homemade foods. Preparing large amount of food is a breeze when you use a food processor, reducing the seemingly endless preparation times for dishes such as vegetables soups and casseroles. A food processor can reduce your chopping, blending, and mixing time by as much as 90 percent. It can also process nuts and seeds into various consistencies. Look for a model with a minimum capacity of 8 to 10 cups (1.9 to 2.3 L) and that comes with both sharp- and soft-edged S-blades, as well as shredding and slicing wheels. The S-blade is useful for making dishes such as hummus or homemade pesto which require mixing, mincing, fine and coarse chopping, and blending; for emulsifying ingredients into salad dressing; and for grinding dry ingredients, such as nuts, seeds, grains, and dried tortillas, into powders.

Electric Blender A high-speed blender is useful for mixing, blending, and grinding. Use it for blending smoothies and shakes, making soups, and achieving the desired degree of smoothness when blending nuts, making pates, or liquefying vegetables.

Handheld Blender This low-cost appliance is great for blending soup while it's still in the pot, as well as whipping cream and beating eggs. Because there is no beaker to wash—unlike a countertop blender—this version saves you time and effort.

Juicer A juice extractor is one of the most convenient ways to get maximum nutrients from fresh fruits and vegetables. The juices extracted from fresh, raw vegetables and fruits furnish all the cells and tissues of the body with minerals, vitamins, and nutritional enzymes in a form that's readily digested and assimilated. We should drink fresh juices daily to nourish our cells and alkalize the body's pH levels.

Some juice extractors have additional blades that enable them to chop and grind food, allowing you to prepare dishes such as nut butters and milks and fruit sorbets. Some of the best brands to look for: Green Star, which is capable of juicing all types of produce, including green leafy vegetables (even grasses), and can homogenize nuts and seeds for patés; the Champion Juicer, which is great for carrots and other vegetables; and the Omega 8002.

Coffee Grinder or Spice Mill A coffee grinder can be used to grind small amounts of whole spices, flaxseeds, and nuts. It's best to grind only the amounts you need for daily use. Flaxseeds and nuts contain delicate omega-3 and omega-6 oils that can easily spoil or turn rancid when stored for any length of time.

Dehydrator Food dehydrators are an excellent product for preserving food enzymes. They work by drying food at low temperatures, usually between 85°F and 115°F (29°C and 46°C), which keeps the enzymes and nutrients intact. Technically, the food is still "raw," because food dehydrating merely extracts the moisture, allowing the food to be better preserved.

Using a dehydrator, you can make crisp crackers and chips, dried fruits and vegetables, fruit leather, protein-rich jerky, and veggie sandwich wraps. (To create a veggie wrap, simply place a piece of kale or chard in the dehydrator for a few minutes, and you have the wrap for any salad or sandwich filling.) You can also make more complex raw treats such as granola, crispy raw almonds and nuts, and sprouted grain crackers. A dehydrator is great for making healthy dehydrated snacks to stock your refrigerator or pantry—just remember that dehydrated foods are still raw and should be eaten within a short time. The Excalibur Dehydrator company manufactures one of the best models on the market.

Wok   A wok is one of the most useful cooking devices and has been used in China for centuries. The wok has the special ability to cook food quickly, so that it retains almost all its nutritional elements. Vegetables most commonly cooked in a wok are carrots, bamboo sprouts, beans (including snap or green beans and soy beans), broccoli, and mushrooms. Using a wok, you can sauté, stew, deep-fry, steam, or stir-fry a meal in just a few minutes. Woks are unbeatable for cooking a bunch of ingredients in a single pan.

Slow Cooker   When you walk in the door after a long day, the last thing you want to do—or have time for—is chop vegetables for dinner. A slow cooker can help by having dinner ready when you arrive, and it's excellent for preparing soups, stews, and casseroles. Simply chop your vegetables and combine them in the cooker with other ingredients, such as grains, herbs, spices, and meat or poultry if desired, and leave them to cook slowly throughout the day. Meals prepared this way are delicious, because the flavors have had time to blend and develop. You can also stock the pot at night with fruits, vegetables, or grains for a healthy, hearty breakfast.

Rice Cooker   Brown rice, buckwheat, and quinoa are all delicious and good for you, and a rice cooker is invaluable for preparing them perfectly. Measure, switch on, and prepare the rest of your dinner. When the timer sounds, the grain is done. You can also prepare fresh warm rice for breakfast by doing the setup overnight.

Healthy Cooking Basics

There are many healthy diets, including macrobiotic, vegan and vegetarian, raw (living) food,

low-carbohydrate, and Ayurvedic, to name a few. It's up to you to find an approach that works best for your metabolism and your lifestyle. The common denominators in all healthy diets and eating regimes is that they rely on natural, home-cooked, genuine-food meals, are devoid of artificial colors and flavors, trans fats, and sugar, and are loaded with phytonutrients, fiber, and good fats.

A Few Words About Meat

There are philosophical and health reasons both for and against consuming factory farmed meats. Moral considerations aside, eating meat raises a number of safety issues. These include the use of harmful antibiotics, growth hormones, and pesticide dips in meat production. The chief problem with eating meat is that cultivated meat is not like the meat from wild animals that fed our ancestors. Livestock animals are given hormones and antibiotics, fed a grain diet to fatten them up (resulting in meat that is higher in saturated fat and toxins), and generally unhealthy. The healthiest meats are from animals raised organically and allowed to graze on grass instead of grain. Grass-fed animals are able to convert the phytonutrients, enzymes, and minerals from grass into lean protein and essential fatty acids.

Meat tends to be a staple in our diet—but it is not always healthy to give it such a prominent place. The main problem is that most meat cultivated today is not like the wild animals on which our ancestors subsisted. Those animals—deer and moose—were free-ranging and therefore much leaner. Moreover, they were not force-fed grains and antibiotics to fatten them up. Modern practices have increased the fat content in animals from about 5 percent to five or six times that amount, causing an equally sizeable impact on our health.

Meats are also the highest acid-ash producing foods. Fruits and vegetables (with very few exceptions) are very alkalizing to our pH. Recall that an alkaline pH is consistent with good health and that we become sick when our body's pH levels are too acidic. The highest acid-producing foods are meats, poultry, and fish, followed by dairy products, eggs, cereals, and grains. By reducing your consumption of high-protein, acid-producing foods, your internal environmental conditions are primed for optimum health.

If you choose to make meat a regular part of your diet, however, you should follow these guidelines:

1. Eat meat in moderation and no more than three times per week. It's not necessary to eat meat every day. Try eating healthier forms of protein, such as quinoa, brown rice, and lentils. The standard American diet, consisting of "meat and two vegetables," is a thing of the past, because we now know it is tied to an abundance of health problems, from digestive upsets to constipation.

2. Don't make meat the centerpiece of the meal. Instead, use vegetables as the star performers and notice how your indigestion and immune system benefit.

3. Try including meat as one element of a dish. For example, add meat to casseroles or large salads, or cook it with vegetables, such as onions, garlic, broccoli, and greens. This way, a little meat goes far in both protecting your health and wallet.

4. Don't make meat as a staple in your diet; reserve it for a special treat or celebration.

5. Eating lots of meat puts added strain on your kidneys and increases your need for hydration. Be sure to drink plenty of clean water both before and after consuming meat.

6. Remember to eat a ratio of 70 percent alkaline-ash to 30 percent acid-ash producing foods. This means that vegetables should make up 70 percent of every meal.

7. Make a point to avoid all cured meats, such as bacon, ham, lunch meats, sausage, and franks, because of their higher amounts of sodium, fat, and cancer-causing chemicals such as nitrites and nitrates.

8. To help cleanse and detoxify the body, go without meat for at least a month and see how you feel. You'll find that your body doesn't need meat at all.

9. Add more fish to your diet, especially salmon, mackerel, herring, and sardines, which deliver omega-3 essential fatty acids. Omega-3s feed your brain and are both anti-inflammatory and heart-friendly. Choose wild over farm-raised fish. Farm-raised fish are raised in pens in the ocean. They aren't allowed much swimming room, are prone to disease (and are therefore fed antibiotics). They have a lower nutritional value than ocean fish, because the pellets they are fed are not the same as the food they would normally eat in the wild—food that they convert into powerful omega-3s.

    Farm-raised fish are also high in mercury. Toxicologists consider mercury one of the most poisonous naturally occurring substances on earth. Because of its tremendous toxicity, it is carefully regulated by the Environmental Protection Agency, the Occupational Safety and Health Administration, and other regulatory bodies. Mercury can also be found in large predatory fish, such as sharks, swordfish, and large tuna (canned tuna is generally made from smaller tuna species that have considerably less mercury contamination than larger tuna). While we do not know the full effect of chronic absorption of even small concentrations of mercury, we do know that mercury exposure can damage many bodily systems, with the nervous, immune, and cardiovascular systems suffering the greatest effects.

10. Avoid eating blackened or charred meat, because it contains harmful free radicals. The best way to ensure that meat retains its enzymes, juices, flavors, and nutrients is to cook it at lower temperatures for longer periods of time. Preferable methods include stir-frying, roasting, and baking.

Excess protein contributes to osteoporosis, over-acidity, and many other common health problems. Protein also plays a key role in the water and sugar balances in the body. It is well known that protein and carbohydrates (sugars) regulate each other. As protein levels in the body rise, so does the need for sugar. This can lead to a cycle of taking in more proteins, followed by more sweet foods and then more protein, and so on, resulting in either a low blood-sugar condition (hypoglycemia) or the more severe conditions of hyperglycemia (a condition in which an excessive amount of glucose circulates in the blood plasma) and diabetes.

As these conditions develop, the stress produced by the high levels of protein and sugar in the body weakens the kidney-adrenal function, which in turn decreases the distribution of fluids in the body. This can lead to dehydration and a buildup of acids in the body. The blood then picks up the acids and transports them to the connective tissues in the body, where they are stored. If too many acids need storing, inflammation and pain develop. This acid overload has been detected in fibromyalgia patients.

Food Preparation Tips and Shortcuts

- Grains and legumes contain phytic acid, an enzyme and mineral inhibitor. Phytic acid can be reduced if you prepare certain foods by first soaking them overnight. Soaking, fermenting, and sprouting are among the most effective techniques for allowing the maximum amount of mineral absorption from foods. When soaking beans and grains, throw away the soaking water and rinse them thoroughly.
- Soak nuts and seeds overnight also and dry them thoroughly. This makes them crunchier and easier to digest. Soaking nuts and seeds helps rid them of enzyme inhibitors, makes them much easier to digest, and makes the fats they contain more available as fatty acids.
- Nuts and seeds can turn rancid and are therefore best refrigerated or even frozen.
- Flour should be kept in the refrigerator or freezer to maintain freshness.
- Fruits, potatoes, tomatoes, onions, and garlic should not be refrigerated. Keep them in a basket in a shady place in the pantry.
- If you're looking for quick-cooking grains, choose millet, quinoa, couscous, and polenta. They require the least amount of cooking time, compared to other grains.
- Fresh herbs keep best when trimmed and placed in a glass of water in the refrigerator.
- Double or triple a recipe and freeze some for future meals or quick snacks.
- Those trying to avoid salt can use low-sodium substitutes, such as kelp, low-sodium tamari, light miso, lemon juice, and celery salt.

Out of the Frying Pan

Because the methods we use to prepare and cook our food can alter the balance between nutrients and anti-nutrients, how we cook is extremely important. Many of the more traditional ways of preparing food are no longer acceptable. For example, frying food in polyunsaturated vegetable oils, such as sunflower, canola oil, and soybean oils, produces lipid hydro-peroxides, which are oxidized molecules that are formed in unsaturated oils when heated at high temperatures. Lipid hydro-peroxides are strong oxidants that produce free radicals in our bodies. As discussed in earlier chapters, these highly reactive chemicals destroy essential fats in food and can damage cells, thereby increasing the

Fats and Oils: Where and How to Use Them

No-Heat Recipes and Salads	Baking	Sautéing	Stir-Frying
Flaxseed oil, pumpkin-seed oil, canola oil, all unrefined vegetable oils	Sesame oil, safflower oil, olive oil, canola oil	Sesame oil, high-oleic safflower oil, olive oil, macadamia nut oil	Coconut oil, peanut oil, macadamia nut oil

risk of cancer, heart disease, and premature aging and destroying the nutrients—vitamins A and E, for example—that protect us from these oxidants.

How much damage is caused by frying depends on the kind of oil used, the temperature at which a food is cooked, and the length of time food is fried. Instead of frying in oil, start with a little water in the pan and add a small amount of oil later on. This reduces the oxidation and rancidity that occurs with frying and helps preserve vital minerals and vitamins in the food. Polyunsaturated oils oxidize most rapidly, particularly when heated; it is therefore best to use them in their raw form. Oils that are predominantly polyunsaturated include walnut, grape-seed, soy, corn, safflower, and sunflower. Coconut oil is saturated and very stable at high heat, so it is recommended for cooking.

Deep frying your food at high temperatures is certainly not as healthful as a light sauté, which is done at a much lower temperature. Steaming, baking, grilling, or boiling is preferable to any form of frying.

You want the right oil for the right cooking job. The less you heat fats and oils, the better. Following are some guidelines to follow when cooking with oils.

Basic Shopping List

Following is a list of food items that serve as the foundation for a healthy pantry. These items supply many of the ingredients you'll need to prepare the recipes in Part II, so stock up for those dishes and any number of nutritious variations.

Grain Products
Brown rice
Bulgur
Gluten-free flours
Rolled Oats
Oatmeal
Popcorn
Quinoa
Wheat germ
Whole-grain bread
Gluten-free or rice crackers
Gluten-free pasta

Vegetables and Fruits
Fresh greens (kale, collards, cabbage, broccoli)
Garlic and onions
Seasonal vegetables
Seasonal fruits
Tomato sauce, paste, and canned tomatoes
Dried fruit (raisins, figs, apricots, dates, prunes)
Frozen vegetables
Frozen fruits

Fats and Oils
Flaxseed oil
Extra-virgin olive oil
Nut oils (walnut, hazelnut)
Toasted sesame oil
Vegetable or lecithin spray
Coconut oil
Grape seed oil

Beans and Lentils
Dried legumes (navy beans, garbanzos, pinto beans, kidney beans, lentils, split peas)
Tofu
Tempeh

Dairy Products (organic or rBGH free)
Butter
Cream
Milk (raw or skim)
Plain yogurt

Nuts, Seeds, and Butters
Nuts (walnuts, pecans, cashews, filberts)
Nut butters
Seeds (almonds, flax, pumpkin, sunflower)
Seed butters (tahini, almond)

Herbs and Spices
Chili powder or other chili
Cinnamon, allspice, nutmeg, cumin
Curry
Fresh parsley, cilantro, basil
Fresh ginger
Fresh and dried oregano, sage, savory, thyme
Mustard, prepared and powdered

Sweeteners
Blackstrap molasses
Barley malt, rice syrup, maple syrup
Honey (locally grown and raw)

Beverages
Leaf and herbal teas
100% fruit and vegetable juices
Cereal-grain beverages, such as dandelion or chicory

Seasonings, Condiments, and Other
Miso
Curry paste
Tamari or soy sauce
Vinegar (apple cider, rice, wine, balsamic)
Seaweed (hijiki, wakame, nori, agar)
Bottled sauces (chili, teriyaki, other)
Vegetable broth powder (without MSG)

Summary

Nutrition is the best means for balancing the body and supplying it with vital nutrients for optimal functioning and longevity.

- Stock your pantry with the building blocks of healthy recipes.
- Avoid unhealthy trans fat, at all costs.
- Clean out all highly processed foods from your pantry, including white-flour and enriched products, high-sugar foods, and foods that contain a lot of preservatives and colorings, have a long shelf life, and have expired.
- Read the label on every product; if it includes an ingredient you don't recognize or understand, don't buy it.
- By organic, antibiotic-free, and hormone-free fresh produce, meat, and dairy.
- Avoid high-fructose corn syrup.
- Increase your fiber intake with fresh fruit and vegetables grown locally, and avoid imported and out-of-season foods grown in artificial environments.
- Familiarize yourself with a healthy shopping list, until it's second nature to shop only for those items on the list.
- Learn which food additives to avoid.
- Make your diet your competitive advantage and your life's work.

CHAPTER 6

BALANCED LIVING PRINCIPLES

When any part of the human body's various systems malfunctions, we call it an imbalance. When imbalance occurs, we start to notice signs of disease and major disorders: low energy, fatigue, poor digestion, excess weight, foggy thinking, aches and pains. Throughout this book we have explored some of the causes that lead to imbalance. The first is something that disturbs your body in some way. The main disturbance is poor diet, although chronic toxicity from external sources, pollution, negative thoughts, spiritual distress, destructive emotions, and other physiological stresses also play a role. When our balance is compromised, so too, is our ability to maintain health, restore vitality, and ward off disease severely compromised.

One of the subtlest forms of bodily imbalance is biochemical. It sneaks up so slowly that we don't see it coming, and it can exist before symptoms present themselves. Eventually, a biochemical imbalance takes its toll. A biochemical deficiency or imbalance is at the root of nearly every disease. However, if you follow the principles of balanced eating and proper nutrition, you will preserve your biochemical balance and are less likely to succumb to sickness and disease. Biochemical balance is a major component, but not the sole contributor, to living a balanced life. Balance also depends on being able to ride out the changes and stresses we all face from time to time. It's about choices, priorities, perspective, and letting go. In this chapter, we'll discuss principles for living your life in balance and how you can restore balance.

Finding Balance

What exactly does it mean, and what does it take, to live in balance in our world today? As we look at our lives, we discover that balance seems to be a central organizing principle of every living system in the universe. The universe exists by keeping opposites in balance, and the universe contained within your body is no exception. Balance equals health, and health equates to energy, mental clarity, smoothly operating body systems, and feeling good. When balanced, we are filled with vitality, enthusiasm, and a sense of purpose. When we have good health, we not only feel good, we can enjoy life. We can be relaxed while watching a movie or on vacation, be energetic at work or play, roll with personal or job-related "punches," and generally find that we wake up in the morning ready to go.

When we are in balance, we experience deep satisfaction. We lose our cravings for sweets and other foods that threaten our inner balance, and we have an appetite for those foods that keep us firmly in balance. We have renewed patience for challenges in our work and relationships. We are clearheaded and can focus on accomplishing our goals. We do not feel rushed and can give our full concentration to the tasks at hand. Simply put, when we live in balance, we feel more in control of our lives on every level—and that's because we are.

For many of us, balance seems to be an elusive quality in our lives, and we have trouble finding it. This is partly because we think it comes from cleaning house or getting up an hour earlier to exercise. We think it's about doing more and juggling as many responsibilities as possible. By trying to keep so much in motion and under our control, we run ourselves ragged. Too often, we end up burned out, relying on stimulants such as sugar, caffeine, nicotine, or worse to keep up the pace and keep ourselves going. Although stimulants seem to offer us a burst of needed energy, they actually drive our system out of balance and force the body to expend more energy to correct the imbalances.

Balance is not a static state that we achieve, once and for all, through the perfect fine-tuning of our daily schedules. Balance is dynamic and constant and exists in a state of equilibrium, in which all facets have equal importance, value, and harmony. In our quest for balance, we encounter the many paradoxes of life, in which everything—every quality, action, or object—is inseparable from its opposite: male and female; night and day; inside and outside; and so on. Both sides must be maintained and supported, as we learn to dance among them, while staying grounded in

flexibility. Balance is essentially about the wholeness in which all opposites and complementary forces find their resolution.

Mindfulness as a Way to Create Balance

One way in which to begin living a more balanced life relates to the way in which we look at life, or our viewpoint. In their book, *Living in Balance*, psychologists Joel and Michelle Levey explain that we should view our journey through life as a walk on a tightrope "stretched across the vastness of space." From this perspective, they claim, life becomes a laboratory, in which to learn how to walk in balance. They describe two primary states of being: one is walking in balance (staying on the rope), and the other is tumbling (mindless, fearful, and out of control). To some degree, they say, we are always either walking mindfully and fully present on our rope or mindlessly tumbling. By recognizing, or becoming *mindful*, that you are tumbling, you are already moving toward balance and you land back on the rope. The trick is not to get more stressed or anxious about tumbling, because this only leads to becoming more out of balance. The name of the game is as much about knowing when you are tumbling as knowing when you are in balance—in other words, to have the presence of mind to recognize when you are in balance and when you are not.

The number one skill for cultivating a balanced way of living, according to the Levys, is *mindfulness*. Through mindfulness, we can develop an internal guidance system that helps us to notice when we're veering off the course of balance, so we can self-correct and find our way back on track. It's certainly not about being perfect, because a quest for perfection only adds pressure. Rather, it is all about learning—learning to recognize the signs that tell us we are off course (or off balance) and gently getting ourselves back on course and in balance. It becomes a life lesson in the art of fine-tuning, similar to that used with a well-tuned instrument, whose most harmonious sounds depend on the strings being neither too tight nor too loose. Through heightened awareness and mindful practice, we sharpen our skills and grow our confidence to a point at which the journey through life becomes one of creative expression, joy, wonder, and discovery.

Relaxation Techniques for Balancing Fibromyalgia Symptoms

Extensive research has shown positive results for fibromyalgia patients from the regular practice of techniques that bring about a *relaxation response* (RR), which decreases the responsiveness of the sympathetic nervous system. The quieting of the sympathetic nervous system is the opposite of the fight-or-flight response and is the essence of relaxation. In addition to the immediate results of decreasing heart rate, blood pressure, breath rate, and oxygen consumption, regular practice over a month or more seems to lead to a change in how the body responds to adrenaline. Research suggests that regularly practicing relaxation response techniques can lead to a reduction in anxiety and depression and an enhanced ability to cope with life stressors.

Relaxation techniques improve overall health and lifestyle balance in the following ways:

- Fewer physical symptoms, such as headaches and back pain
- Increased energy
- Better control of your emotions, such as anger or frustration
- Improved concentration
- Greater ability to handle problems
- More efficiency in day-to-day activities

The relaxation response differs from the feelings we experience listening to music or enjoying a hobby, which are fairly temporary. The relaxation response creates immediate, as well as long-term, physiological changes in the body that become

even more pronounced and effective, once a person has been specifically trained in RR and the longer they practice the techniques. It's a process that lessens the wear and tear of life's challenges on your mind and body.

Relaxation techniques usually involve refocusing your attention on something calming and increasing awareness of your body. There are several types of relaxation techniques, which we will discuss in more detail below. An important first step, however, to learning or applying any of these relaxation techniques is proper breathing. Improper breathing contributes to anxiety, panic attacks, depression, muscle tension, headaches, and fatigue. As you learn to be aware of your breathing patterns and practice slowing and normalizing your breaths with deep abdominal breathing, your mind will quiet and your body will relax. As a natural response, you will reduce the muscle tension and anxiety that accompany stress-related symptoms or thoughts. Deep or abdominal breathing is the easiest and surest way to elicit the relaxation response.

The Health Benefits of Deep Abdominal Breathing

Deep abdominal breathing is important, because it increases our vitality and promotes relaxation. We have moved away from healthy abdominal breathing, due to years of stress, anxiety, and tension, which impede our breathing. When we try to practice deep breathing, most of us tend to do the opposite: We suck in our bellies and raise our shoulders. This is shallow breathing. When we breathe fully and deeply, the diaphragm moves farther down in to the abdomen, allowing our lungs to expand more completely into the chest cavity. With each deep breath, more oxygen is taken in and more carbon dioxide is released.

Deep abdominal breathing can have a powerful influence on our health and well-being, because it helps turn on our parasympathetic nervous system—our relaxation response. When our breathing is full and deep, the diaphragm moves through its entire range of motion—downward to massage the liver, stomach, and other organs and tissues below it, and upward to massage the heart. In deep abdominal breathing, the diaphragm's downward and upward movements help to massage and detoxify our inner organs, promote blood flow and peristalsis, and pump the lymph more efficiently through our lymphatic system. The lymphatic system is an important part of our immune system and benefits greatly from the movements of breathing. By practicing deep abdominal breathing, we help to balance our central nervous system and reduce the amount of stress in our lives, which yields positive results for our overall health.

Deep Breathing Technique

1. Lie on your back on a firm surface, with your spine straight.

2. Scan your body for tension.

3. Place one hand on your abdomen and one hand on your chest.

4. Inhale deeply and slowly through your nose into your abdomen, to push up your hand as much as feels comfortable. Your chest should move only slightly and only with your abdomen. Be sure to do this slowly, over 8 to 10 seconds.

5. Hold your breath for a second or two. When you feel comfortable with step 4, exhale through your mouth, making a quiet, relaxing, whooshing sound, as you gently expel the air. Continue to take long, slow, deep breaths that raise and lower your abdomen. Notice yourself becoming more and more relaxed as you focus on your breathing.

6. Continue deep breathing for about 5 to 10 minutes at a time, once or twice a day. If you find yourself getting dizzy, then you are overdoing it and should slow down. Try to extend your sessions for as long as possible, to increase the relaxation benefits.

7. You can also imagine yourself in a peaceful situation such as a warm gentle ocean or beautiful garden.

8. After each deep-breathing session, scan your body again for any tension. Compare the tension you felt at the beginning to how you feel at the end of the session.

9. When you have learned to relax yourself using deep abdominal breathing, practice any time of the day, when you feel like it or when you feel yourself getting tense.

   In time, you will learn to quickly identify any stress reaction or tension in your body and take immediate steps to alleviate it through deep breathing.

I recommend practicing deep breathing techniques daily as a way to help balance your energies. Breathing not only unleashes life's energy—it also provides a healing pathway into the deepest recesses of our being and allows us to connect to our wholeness and inner healing powers.

Progressive Muscle Relaxation

The technique of progressive muscle relaxation involves isolating one muscle group, creating tension for 8 to 10 seconds, and then letting the muscle relax and release the tension. Through repeated practice, you quickly learn to recognize and distinguish the feelings associated with a tensed muscle and a relaxed muscle. With this simple knowledge, you can induce physical muscular relaxation at the earliest signs of tension accompanying stress and anxiety. Deep muscle relaxation is incompatible with anxiety, because the habit of responding with one blocks the habit of responding with the other.

Progressive muscle relaxation helps people with sleep problems get a good night's sleep. Excellent results have also been reached in treating muscle spasms, back and neck pain, anxiety, depression, fatigue, high blood pressure, and irritable bowel syndrome. Most people do not realize which of their muscles are chronically tense. Progressive muscle relaxation is a way to identify particular muscles and muscle groups and to distinguish between sensations of tension and deep relaxation. All you need to begin undoing what stress has done to your body is to learn to systematically relax your muscles.

The progressive muscle relaxation technique goes as follows:

1. Sit or lie comfortably in a quiet room, where you won't be disturbed for at least 10 to 15 minutes. Wear loose clothing and remove your shoes.

2. Slowly inhale and exhale, using deep breaths, closing your eyes as you do so. Feel yourself relax.

3. As you let the rest of your body relax, clench your fists and bend them back at the wrist, tighter and tighter, as you briefly hold the tension. Feel the tension in your wrists and forearm, then relax and let go.

4. Gradually work your way down the body to your chest, stomach, back and spine, buttocks, legs, and feet, until you reach your toes. Continue tensing and relaxing each area, alternating between the left and right sides, until your entire body has been worked on progressively.

By the time you finish, your whole body will feel more relaxed. Your heart rate will slow down, your blood pressure will drop, and your breathing will become regular and deep. You will find, over time, that your muscles will gradually become even more relaxed than when you started. You will also notice mood changes—you become more calm, refreshed, and balanced. You will enjoy a number of other health benefits, such as healthy digestion, as well.

Guided Deep Relaxation: Yoga Nidra

Yoga nidra is a powerful, ancient form of guided meditation that induces relaxation and healing of the body, mind and spirit.

You will benefit from this practice if you suffer from:

- Chronic pain
- Fibromyalgia
- Chronic fatigue syndrome
- Depression
- PTSD (Post-Traumatic Stress Disorder)
- Insomnia
- Anxiety
- Restlessness
- Stress-related disorders

Regular practice of yoga nidra is a healthy habit that rests, restores, and renews the body, mind, and spirit, offering the opportunity to process and release the accumulated stress and tension that cause physical and mental illness.

Regular practitioners of yoga nidra report that they experience better sleep, less physical pain, and more emotional ease and well-being. It comes from the tantric yoga tradition and its practice is simple: all you do is lie down, listen, and receive as you are guided through all layers of your being to relax, heal, and rejuvenate your body mind and spirit. Tantric is a Sanskrit word for expand, extend, or manifest. I have designed several yoga nidra sessions especially to relieve chronic pain and insomnia for people with fibromyalgia. You can enjoy a free introductory session or learn more on my website.

Creative Visualization and Guided Imagery

You have probably heard it said that your thoughts become your reality—in other words, you are what you think you are. The power of your imagination to create emotional states is undeniable. For example, if you think sad or anxious thoughts, it follows that you begin to feel unhappy or tense. By the same token, to counter these feelings, you should refocus your mind on positive, healing images. The same is true when you focus only on the negative aspect of a particular illness or problem—that aspect grows in importance and becomes more problematic. To heal and find resolution to problems, you must first turn your attention toward healing and becoming a part of the solution. Positive imagery is certainly a better use of your mental energy than imagining all the bad things that can happen! The more you keep your thoughts anchored in healing and on finding solutions to problems, the more cooperation and opportunity you meet because your mind is attuned to the positive.

Creative visualization (often referred to as guided imagery) is a method that asks you to imagine yourself in a particular scene leading to a desired action or outcome. It is a potent technique for reducing stress, especially when combined with physical relaxation methods, such as deep breathing. Research has shown that stimulating the brain through visualization and imagery may have a direct effect on both the endocrine and nervous systems, which leads to changes in immune-system function.

The idea behind using imagery and visualization to reduce stress is that you use your imagination to re-create and enjoy a relaxing situation. Guided imagery, as its name implies, guides a person or group with words designed to create images for various purposes, such as relaxation, stress management, and healing—both mental and physical.

The more intensely you imagine the situation, and the more senses you employ while imagining, the more relaxing the experience becomes.

Guided imagery teaches you to relax and find comfort in any situation, whether you are sick or healthy. It can reduce anxiety by 65 percent or more, and it has been shown to decrease pain and bring a person to a state of tranquility in a matter of minutes. Imagery can help you tap into inner strengths and find hope, courage, patience, perseverance, love, and other qualities that help you cope with, transcend, and overcome almost any illness.

Visualization and guided imagery are effective tools that have been used successfully for combating a variety of health issues, including:

- Stress-related and physical illnesses, including muscles spasms and chronic pain
- Headaches
- Anxiety
- Pain
- Post-traumatic stress
- Smoking
- Addictions
- Obesity
- Anger
- Insomnia

Visualization and guided imagery are practiced and studied in cancer and pain centers throughout the country. To use visualization as a relaxation tool, imagine a scene, place, or event that feels safe, peaceful, restful, beautiful, and happy. Bring as many of your senses as possible into play—for example, the warmth of the sun, the smell of your favorite flowers, the sounds of running water and birds, or the taste of a refreshing cool drink on a hot day. Use the imagined place as your special retreat from stress and pressure.

The technique might run as follows:

1. Loosen your clothing and remove your shoes, lie down in a quiet comfortable place, and gently close your eyes. Be sure that it's a place in which you won't be interrupted.

2. Carefully chosen music can be very useful in creating the right atmosphere and setting the right mood. The music should be soothing and may incorporate natural sounds, such as birds or falling rain. Soft lighting, such as candles or small lanterns, is preferable.

3. Aromatherapy oils or incense can add to the ambience but should not be overpowering. The scent of lavender is particularly relaxing.

4. Begin with several minutes of deep breathing exercises, to become more conscious of your body and breath. This will relax you in preparation for your visualization and imagery session. Be aware that it takes practice to imagine with all your senses; for example, some people have difficulty seeing colors, or imagining a smell, taste, sound, or sensation. At first, it is enough just to imagine that you are surrounded by green trees or that a light breeze is blowing.

5. As you relax, scan your body, seeking tension in specific muscles. Relax those muscles as much as possible, using deep breathing.

6. Begin to form mental sense impressions. Involve all your senses: sight, hearing, smell, touch, and taste. For instance, imagine a deserted beach with waves rolling in gently, blue sky, sand between your toes, the smell of the ocean. Add more sounds, smells, and other senses as you relax into your images; for example, bring in seagulls and birdcalls, waves crashing on the shore, and so on.

7. Use affirmation. Repeat short, positive statements that affirm your ability to relax. Use the present tense and avoid negatives, such as, "I am not tense," in favor of positives, such as,

"I am letting go of tension."

Other examples of positive affirmations:

My mind is calm.

I am calm and relaxed in every situation.

My thoughts are under my control.

I am surrounded by love.

Every day, in every way, I am getting better and better.

Use visualization or guided imagery up to three times a day. A typical session may last from fifteen minutes to half an hour or more, depending on content and objectives. Visualization practice is easiest in the morning and at night, while you lie in bed. After some practice, you will be able to visualize in any location: on the bus, in the doctor's waiting room, before going into a meeting, or during a visit to the dentist. Most importantly, visualization and guided imagery give you a measure of control over your life. No matter the circumstances, you will be able to relax easily, calm down, and sleep better.

Meditation and Mindfulness

Meditation has been used for healing for centuries. Meditating a few minutes each day has been proven to reduce stress, and it can improve your mood and view of life as well. Although there are various meditation methods, they all have one thing in common: They focus on quieting the mind.

It's important to understand that we are not talking about reaching a higher level or state of mind (although many people use meditation for just that reason). Quite simply, the aim of meditation is to tame our mind by using the aforementioned technique of mindfulness. Meditation is used to overcome anxiety, agitation, and all sorts of habitual thought patterns, so that we can sit with a calm and focused mind and experience life in the here and now.

Often, our thoughts dwell on something that happened in the past or are fixated on something we want to happen in the future—two major sources of chronic stress. When we're lost in the past or projecting into the future, we fail to pay attention to what's going on around us, and we miss out on life as it unfolds. When we practice meditation and being mindful, we keep our attention anchored in the present. In this way, we are completely absorbed in the fabric of life, the fabric of the moment. We may have memories of the past and ideas about the future, but it is the present situation that we are experiencing. This allows us to be spontaneous and to experience our life fully.

We begin meditation by using our breath as the basis of our focus and our mindfulness. The nature of the mind is such that it does not want to stay fixed. A parade of thoughts, ideas, questions, and concepts will present themselves and try to interfere with the meditation. Our breath brings us back to the present moment. Every time we have a distracting thought, we note to ourselves that we're thinking and return to following the breath. If, for instance, we wonder what's for dinner, we simply label it "thinking."

Each time you realize that your mind has drifted away from your breath, gently acknowledge it and let it go. By repeating this moment of awareness, this technique of mindfulness (which consists of noticing stray thoughts and then refocusing the attention back to your breath), surprising realizations become apparent:

- It isn't necessary to think about every thought that pops into your head. You have the power to choose what you think about.
- You will learn how to remain calm in any situation.
- Most diseases develop from a state of discord between mind and body. Meditation brings your body, mind, emotions, and spirit—every facet of human existence—into harmony, like a symphony orchestra.

- Because no one can think two thoughts simultaneously, it is impossible to worry, fear, or hate when your mind is focused in a meditative state. During meditation, the aim is to be fully present in the moment, where there is no fear, worry, or negative emotion.
- Even the strongest emotion will become manageable if you concentrate on the sensations in your body and not the content of the thought that produced the emotion.

As a result of practicing meditation, your heart rate and breathing slow, your blood pressure normalizes, you use oxygen more efficiently, and you sweat less. Your adrenal glands produce less cortisol, adrenaline, and noradrenaline, you make more positive hormones, your body ages at a slower rate, and your immune function improves. Your mind also clears and your creativity increases. People who meditate regularly find it easier to give up life-damaging habits, such as smoking, drinking, and drugs.

Regular meditation also:

- Leads to a deeper level of relaxation
- Decreases muscle tension (and pain caused by tension)
- Helps with chronic conditions, such as allergies, arthritis, and fibromyalgia
- Increases serotonin production, which influences mood and behavior (low levels of serotonin are associated with depression, obesity, insomnia and headaches)
- Decreases depression and anxiety
- Improves learning ability and memory
- Increases feelings of vitality and rejuvenation
- Increases emotional stability
- Increases self-confidence

Other recommended relaxation techniques to use include:

- Yoga
- Music
- Exercise

- Tai chi
- Massage
- Hypnosis

Explore as many ways to relax as possible, to discover the ones that work best for you and your lifestyle.

Mindful Eating

To eat mindfully is to eat in a conscious and supportive manner, using our body's cues to guide us in determining when, what, and how much we need for satisfaction and well-being. When practiced regularly, mindful eating can increase awareness of our thoughts, feelings, and motivations, which are important elements in our quest for balanced living and optimum health.

Eating to achieve a balance of physical nourishment, mental relaxation, and emotional harmony involves the interplay of many factors, and our goals can be undermined when we let certain patterns develop or lose our view of food as a way to nourish every aspect of our health. Preparing and anticipating a wholesome meal and enjoying its aromas, colors, and tastes are delightful ways to add pleasure to our daily routine, while taking care of and nurturing ourselves. Let's take a brief look at the healthful ways we can approach food and our relationship with it.

Create a Peaceful Setting

To receive proper nourishment, we must be receptive. If we eat on the run or while doing other things, we do not permit ourselves to pay attention to the whole process of eating—chewing, tasting, and swallowing our food. This often leads to difficulties with digestion and absorption. It's important to give our full attention to the preparation of a meal. If you prepare meals with a nourishing spirit and an attitude of appreciation, it is likely that the person eating them will experience those qualities, too. Alternately, when a meal is prepared amid stress and frustration, it takes on an entirely

different "flavor."

Strive to create a tranquil environment when cooking and eating a meal. If you find that you are particularly sensitive to the presence of others or are easily upset, it might be best to eat in peace by yourself or with those who also prefer to eat quietly.

Eat Slowly

Take small bites and savor the color, taste, and texture of the food. Avoid watching television or reading while eating. Focus on the experience, so you notice each food's flavor, texture, and aroma. Set your fork down between bites, and don't pick it up until you are done chewing and swallowing. If you are very hungry, this can be difficult. Take deep breaths to help slow down your eating.

Listen to Your Appetite

The first rule of eating: Eat when you are hungry. Hunger tells us that our body has digested and used the last food we consumed and is ready for more. Learn to listen to your body's needs and to know when you are truly hungry. Pay attention to the emotional triggers that prompt you to eat out of boredom, anxiety, or the need for oral gratification rather than a genuine physical feeling of hunger. Disordered eating may reflect unbalanced states of emotional distress, such as depression or loneliness. When you find yourself eating in response to boredom or an emotional state, substitute a pleasurable activity, such as a walk, a conversation with a friend, or a hobby. If you feel you eat more often for emotional reasons than for physical nourishment, you might find counseling helpful.

Enjoy Your Food

When you eat, it's important to savor your food with your eyes and nose, as well as your mouth. Digestive juices begin flowing from the moment we see or smell food that's appealing, so using and being aware of all your senses enhances your enjoyment and helps you feel more satisfied. Make mealtimes special. Mealtimes are opportunities to nurture yourself and provide sustenance for the body, mind, and spirit. What you eat affects how you think and how you feel; they are intimately connected. Give yourself the gift of the highest-quality whole foods, and every aspect of your body, mind, and spirit will reward you.

This chapter has introduced you to many different ways of reducing anxiety, managing stress, and making each day calm and peaceful. I recommend trying each exercise at least once, to find the combination that works for you. Doing the exercise you most enjoy should take no longer than 20 to 30 minutes, depending on how much time you wish to spend. Ideally, you should do the exercises daily. Over time, they will help you gain insight into yourself in ways that may surprise you. You will discover how to turn negative feelings and beliefs into positive, self-nurturing ones. Your confidence will grow, as you master the ability to cope with stress and anxiety. As for your health, your symptoms will diminish, and you will feel stronger and more resilient, as you gain control over your life.

Summary

- A biochemical deficiency or imbalance is at the root of nearly every disease.
- Balance is essentially about wholeness, in which all opposites and complementary forces find their resolution.
- Balance is dynamic and constant. It is a state of equilibrium in which all sides have equal importance, value, and harmony.
- Through mindfulness, we can develop an internal guidance system that helps us recognize when we're heading off a balanced course.
- Relaxation techniques can improve overall health and lifestyle balance by evoking the relaxation response.
- Deep abdominal breathing, progressive muscle relaxation, visualization and guided imagery, meditation, and mindfulness are powerful allies to balanced nutrition and can be used to restore balance to your life.
- A holistic, mindful strategy that includes dietary improvements and is supported by relaxation therapies can overcome fibromyalgia and provide you with a richer life experience, by giving you an intimate connection to your body and a sense of personal responsibility for your health and well-being.

PART II

WINNING THE BATTLE THROUGH FOOD

INTRODUCTION: UNDERSTANDING THE RECIPES

The Health Facilitators Chart

Following are some guidelines for the recipes. For your convenience, and to make it easier to balance your food choices for optimum nutrition selections, each recipe has been rated to indicate the level of each of these health facilitators: macronutrients (protein, fat, and carbohydrates), enzymes, antioxidants, and fiber.

Each health facilitator is rated—in chart form—by its level of nutrient density, using the following rating system:

- None—recipe contains no useful quantity
- Low—provides small amounts
- Moderate—provides average levels
- High—provides better-than-average levels
- Very High—provides optimum levels

Fine-Tuning the Ratings

At the beginning of each recipe chapter are detailed instructions and suggestions to help you increase or decrease the rating of any of the health facilitators in a particular recipe. Suggestions for a leafy green salad, for example, may include the following:

- To increase protein levels, add any of the following ingredients: hard-boiled egg, tuna, salmon, chicken, or feta cheese.
- To increase fatty acid levels, add any of the following ingredients: black olives, avocado, or feta cheese.

- To increase fiber and antioxidant levels, add more vegetables. Adding brown rice, lentils, garbanzo beans, quinoa, and other grains and legumes will increase the fiber, protein, and carbohydrate levels.
- To increase enzymes levels, add any raw or live vegetable, or squeeze fresh lemon or lime juice directly onto the salad.

These recipes are good starting points. By understanding the health facilitator categories and nutrient densities of the foods in each recipe, you can make adjustments by adding or deleting ingredients to best serve your metabolism and to achieve optimally balanced meals. By working with these recipes and following the principles outlined in Chapter 4, you will become an expert at listening to your body and fine-tuning these and other recipes to your particular health needs. The macronutrient chart on page 53, and the Glycemic Index chart on page 60, will assist you in this process.

"Raw" Recipes

Finally, you will see that certain recipes have been designated *raw*, which means that the dish requires no cooking. Many who have embraced a raw-food diet have found relief from a host of conditions, including fibromyalgia. Other conditions that can be alleviated by a raw (living) food diet are diabetes, acne, migraines, joint pain, asthma, high blood pressure, high cholesterol, hypoglycemia, colitis and diverticulitis, arthritis, allergies, depression, anxiety and mood swings, heartburn, gas and bloating, obesity, menopausal symptoms, chronic fatigue, and cancer.

New-to-You Ingredients

The recipes include a number of ingredients with which you may not be familiar. Following is a breakdown of those ingredients, with an explanation of what they are, why they're beneficial, and where you can buy them.

Himalayan Crystal Salt

This salt is hand-mined from the Himalayan Mountains with respect for the environment, the workers, and its inherent bioenergetic properties. It restores the body's alkaline and electrolyte balance, and it contains eighty-four minerals and trace elements essential to the body's health and well-being. It yields positive changes in respiratory, circulatory, organ, connective tissue, and nervous system functions. It can be found in selected health food and vitamin stores or purchased online.

Pure-Pressed Extra-Virgin Olive Oil

This is the highest-quality and most nutritious olive oil. It is collected from the first pressing of the fruit without the use of heat (called cold-pressing), which helps retain the maximum nutrition content. It is heavy and rich, with a darkish yellow-green color and a fruity-peppery aroma. Both oils contain the essential fatty acid, alpha linolenic acid, and are available at supermarkets.

Flaxseed Oil

Derived from the seeds of the flax plant, flaxseed oil is a rich source of omega-3 essential fatty acids and contains lignans (compounds known for their cancer-fighting properties). Flaxseed oil can turn rancid if not refrigerated, and it requires special packaging to protect it from heat, light, and oxygen. You should be able to find flaxseed oil in health food stores and the organic section of most supermarkets.

Rapadura

Rapadura is the commercial name for dehydrated cane sugar juice, which people in India have used for thousands of years. It is rich in minerals, particularly silica and iron. Rapadura has a great flavor and closely mimics sugar in chemical properties. It yields wonderful results with baking—just be careful not to overdo it, because rapadura is a concentrated sweetener. If you have sugar balance problems, use it sparingly and with care. You can purchase rapadura in most health food stores.

Coconut Butter

Coconut butter is the solid form of coconut oil. It is a tasty, healthy, naturally saturated vegetable product. Coconut butter is very stable, making it ideal for sautéing and baking. Coconut oil contains "good" fat (50 percent lauric acid), and it does not elevate your "bad" cholesterol level (LDL). Slightly lower in calories than most vegetable oils, coconut oil and butter can be found in the organic section of most supermarkets, in health food stores, or online.

Carob Powder

Carob is known as the healthy alternative to chocolate, because it is free of the stimulants found in chocolate: caffeine and theobromine. Carob is naturally sweet, so products that use it generally contain substantially less sugar than their chocolate counterparts. Carob powder can be substituted for cocoa powder in any recipe and is available at most supermarkets.

Kombu Seaweed

This dark green sea vegetable comes from the kelp family and is used frequently in Japanese cooking. It adds flavor to soups, stews, and almost any dish that requires a salty taste. A rich source of protein, calcium, iodine, magnesium, iron, and folate, kelp has been linked to low rates of breast cancer in Japanese women. You can find kombu in health food stores and Asian markets.

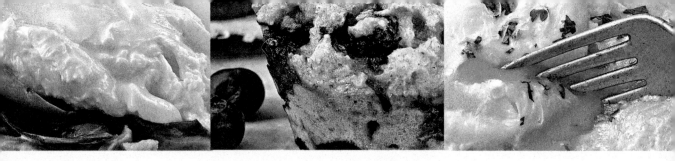

CHAPTER 7

GREAT BEGINNINGS

Berry Buzz Smoothie (RAW)

Power up with protein from the tofu and rice protein powder, and then supercharge this smoothie with bee pollen, barley, or wheat grass for a shot of antioxidants and enzymes to start your day. Adding D-ribose (Corvalen) into the mix ensures that you have sustained energy for many hours. For more on D-ribose, see note below and page 243.

INGREDIENTS

10 raw almonds or 5 raw macadamia nuts
5 ounces (140 g) (½ package) tofu
2 cups (290 g) fresh or frozen fruit
  or berries
1 cup (235 ml) pure water
1 scoop or 2 heaping tablespoons (16 g)
  rice protein powder
1½ teaspoons (3 to 4 g) D-ribose (Corvalen)
1 tablespoon (15 ml) olive oil or flaxseed oil

Optional:

1 to 2 tablespoons (1 to 2 g) bee pollen,
  powdered barley, or wheat grass
½ to 1 cup (75 to 150 g) ice cubes

Yield: 1 serving

Grind nuts in a coffee grinder or food processor.

Combine all ingredients in a blender until smooth and creamy. Pour into a large glass and serve cold.

Did You Know?

D-ribose is a carbohydrate, or naturally occurring sugar, used by all living cells and is an essential component in our body's energy production. It is part of the building blocks that form DNA and RNA molecules. Adding D-ribose to this smoothie ensures you have sustained energy for many hours.

Health Facilitators	Nutrient Density Rating
Protein	Very High
Fat	Moderate
Carbohydrate	Moderate
Enzymes	High
Antioxidants	High
Fiber	Moderate

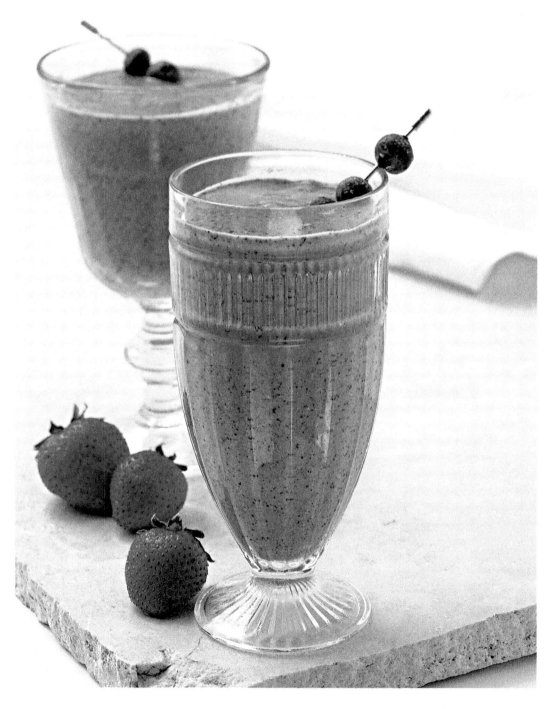

Cleansing Fig Smoothie (RAW)

Delight your senses with the exotic tastes of figs, mango, and coconut, while helping improve intestinal function. Figs are rich in potassium, calcium, phosphorus, magnesium, iron, and copper, and this entire blend of power foods supports blood formation and delivers an energy boost. Add bee pollen, barley, or wheat grass for a shot of extra antioxidants and enzymes to start your day.

INGREDIENTS
¼ cup (42 g) flaxseeds
5 dried or fresh figs
Spring water
2 cups (475 ml) fresh apple juice
1 scoop or 2 heaping tablespoons (16 g) rice protein powder
1½ teaspoons D-ribose (Corvalen)
½ mango
½ avocado
2 tablespoons (28 ml) flaxseed oil
Coconut butter to taste
Ice cubes as needed

Optional
1 to 2 tablespoons (1 to 2 grams) bee pollen, powdered barley, or wheat grass

Yield: 1 serving

Grind flaxseeds in a coffee grinder or food processor. Soak dried figs in spring water for at least 30 minutes. Combine all ingredients in a blender until smooth and creamy. Add ice and coconut butter to taste. Pour into a large glass and serve cold.

Did You Know?
Recently published studies have shown that after supplementing with D-ribose, fibromyalgia and chronic fatigue syndrome (CFS) sufferers enjoyed an average 44 percent increase in energy after only three weeks, and an average overall improvement in quality of life of 30 percent. For more on D-ribose, see page 243.

Health Facilitators	Nutrient Density Rating
Protein	High
Fat	High
Carbohydrate	Moderate
Enzymes	High
Antioxidants	High
Fiber	High

Nut Milk (RAW)

Enjoy this enzyme-packed, nutrient-dense alternative to cow's milk. Enjoy your fresh milk over granola, with dessert, or on its own.

INGREDIENTS

1 cup (145 g) nuts (almonds, pecans, macadamia, or hazelnut) or 1 cup (145g) sesame seeds
1 to 2 cups (235 to 475 ml) spring or filtered water
½ cup (75 g) dried fruit such as figs, dates, or raisins
Dash cinnamon
Piece of cheesecloth or clean nylon stocking

Yield: 2 cups (475 ml)

Soak nuts or seeds in pure water for approximately 12 hours or overnight. Soak dried fruit for 4 to 6 hours; drain and reserve liquid. Place the nuts in a blender and pulverize. Add 1 cup (235 ml) of water gradually, while continuing to blend on high.

Add cinnamon, and additional water or liquid from soaking dried fruit, so that your mixture will have a sufficiently liquid consistency to strain—about 1 cup (145 g) nuts or seeds to 2 cups (475 ml) liquid. Strain through a piece of cheesecloth or nylon stocking.

Nut milk should be stored in a glass container in the refrigerator, and lasts 3 to 4 days.

Note: You can dehydrate the pulp that remains after straining. Simply spread pulp on a Teflex sheet. Dehydrate at 110°F (43°C) for about 8 hours, or until totally dry and flaky. Sprinkle pulp on top of desserts, or use as "flour" in bread recipes.

Health Facilitators	Nutrient Density Rating
Protein	High
Fat	High
Carbohydrate	Low
Enzymes	High
Antioxidants	High
Fiber	High

"Hi-Fibe" Blueberry Muffins

Indulge yourself with 100-percent delicious, high-fiber, protein-packed blueberry muffins. The whole grain and rolled oats will boost your fiber intake, while the berries deliver additional fiber and antioxidants such as vitamin C and vitamin A. Blueberries are plentiful in minerals, such as potassium and calcium, and with the addition of eggs, these muffins provide adequate levels of healthy fat and protein.

INGREDIENTS

½ teaspoon butter for greasing tin
1 cup (120 g) gluten-free flour
1 cup (80 g) rolled oats
1½ teaspoons cinnamon
½ teaspoon gluten-free baking powder
¼ teaspoon baking soda
½ teaspoon Himalayan crystal salt
6 tablespoons (48 g) rice protein powder
¼ cup (60 ml) coconut oil
2 eggs
1 teaspoon stevia extract
   mixed with ½ cup (120 ml) rice milk
2 cups (290 g) fresh or frozen blueberries]
6 dates (chopped)
½ cup (75 g) rasins
1 banana (mashed)
1 cup (100 g) walnuts (chopped)

Yield: 12 muffins

Preheat oven to 400°F (200°C, or gas mark 6) and grease muffin tins with butter. In a large mixing bowl, combine flour, rolled oats, cinnamon, baking powder, baking soda, and salt. Blend protein powder, coconut oil, eggs, stevia extract, and rice milk until smooth. Stir into dry ingredients. Gently fold in blueberries, raisins, and banana. Fill muffin tins to top and bake 18 to 20 minutes. Serve each muffin with 1/3 cup (48 g) fresh berries.

Did You Know?

Stevia extract, which comes from a small plant native to Paraguay and Brazil, is 250 times sweeter than table sugar. Results of short- and long-term studies indicate that it is a safe supplement for the human diet and that it promotes healthy blood sugar levels. You can find stevia in health food stores and some supermarkets.

Health Facilitators	Nutrient Density Rating
Protein	High
Fat	Moderate
Carbohydrate	High
Enzymes	Moderate
Antioxidants	Moderate
Fiber	High

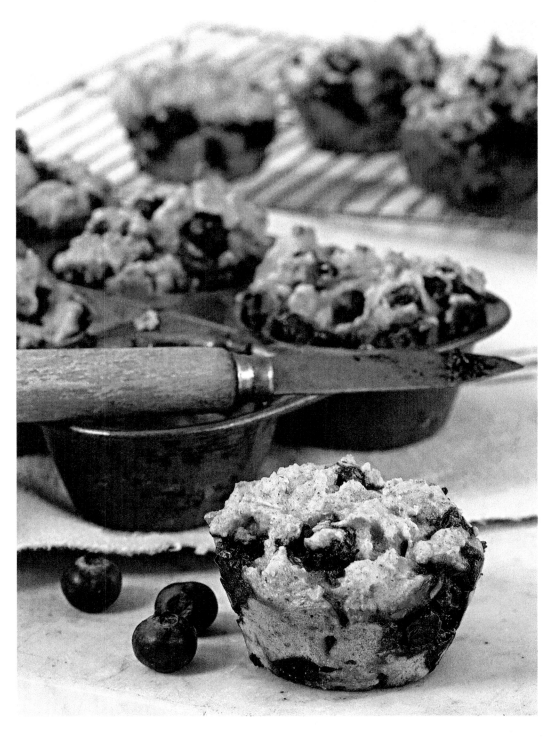

Lively Fresh Fruit over Ground Nuts and Seeds (RAW)

Here's one of the most nutrient-dense, fiber-filled breakfasts you can eat that delivers all the benefits of eating raw. Flaxseeds are high in fiber and omega-3s, which help fight inflammation. Almonds are probably the best all-around nut, because they are available year round, are a leading source of vitamin E, are high in vitamin B, fiber, potassium, protein, phosphorus, and iron, and are a tasty source of calcium.

INGREDIENTS
1 tablespoon (6 g) raw almonds
1 tablespoon (9 g) raw pumpkin seeds
1 tablespoon (9 g) raw sunflower seeds
2 tablespoons (24 g) flaxseeds
½ to 1 cup (115 to 230 g) yogurt
½ to 1 cup (75 to 145 g) chopped fresh seasonal fruit (e.g., berries, peaches, pears, bananas)
1 tablespoon (15 ml) flaxseed oil

Yield: 1 serving

Soak the almonds, pumpkin seeds, and sunflower seeds overnight to enhance their digestibility and increase enzymes. (Note: Do not soak the flaxseeds, because they will swell and become gelatinous, making them much harder to eat.) Place almonds and seeds in a coffee grinder or food processor and blend into a meal-like consistency. Place in a bowl and add yogurt, fruit, and flaxseed oil. Serve immediately.

Did You Know?
Pumpkin seeds are known for their concentration of zinc and their use in treating and preventing male prostate problems. Sunflower seeds, used throughout history to enhance energy, have a number of health-enhancing benefits.

Health Facilitators	Nutrient Density Rating
Protein	High
Fat	Moderate
Carbohydrate	High
Enzymes	Very High
Antioxidants	High
Fiber	Very High

Banana Quinoa Porridge

If you've never tried quinoa for breakfast you're in for a treat. Quinoa is great with the sweet taste of fruit or served with more savory items such as vegetables. It's a dieter's dream because it is satisfying and will fill you up; is high in protein, rich in fiber, and digested slowly; and has a low glycemic index, helping you keep your blood sugar levels stable for hours. Quinoa is a flavorful source of plant-derived calcium, so it helps regulate contraction of the heart and facilitates nerve and muscle function. It's perfect for fighting fibromyalgia pain and also contains impressive amounts of potassium, magnesium, and zinc.

INGREDIENTS
4 cups (692 g) quinoa
1 cup (178 g) pitted and chopped fresh dates
1½ cups (352 ml) filtered water
1 banana
1 teaspoon ground cinnamon
1 teaspoon ground nutmeg

Yield: 6 cups (1110 g)

Soak the quinoa overnight in filtered water and drain the next morning. Soak the dates overnight in the filtered water. Blend the quinoa, dates and their soaking liquid, banana, cinnamon, and nutmeg in an electric blender until smooth. Serve cold or at room temperature.

Health Facilitators	Nutrient Density Rating
Protein	High
Fat	Low
Carbohydrate	Moderate
Enzymes	High
Antioxidants	Moderate
Fiber	High

Greenies Delight Quiche

This crustless quiche is packed with fiber from broccoli, which is rich in vitamins A, C, and B and minerals such as potassium, calcium, magnesium, and iron. Serve it on a bed of spinach for enzymes and added fiber and for another dose of vitamins A and C, which are good sources of antioxidants to help keep your immune system strong.

INGREDIENTS

1½ cups (110 g) chopped broccoli florets
4 eggs
1 cup (235 ml) organic cream
½ cup (120 ml) pure water
Freshly ground black pepper to taste
Dash cayenne pepper
1 cup (120 g) grated Gruyere, mozzarella, or cheddar cheese
½ cup (50 g) chopped scallions
½ cup (30 g) fresh chopped parsley
1 large bunch (4 cups [120 g]) fresh spinach, washed

Yield: 6 servings

Preheat oven to 350°F (180°C, or gas mark 4). Lightly steam broccoli florets. In a medium bowl, using a fork, whisk eggs, cream, water, black pepper, and cayenne pepper until well blended. Add grated cheese and mix well.

Butter a 9- or 10-inch (23- or 25-cm) pie pan or dish. Scatter broccoli and scallions in the bottom of the pan. Pour in egg and cheese mixture. Place pie pan on a baking sheet and bake 45 to 50 minutes, or until a knife inserted into center comes out clean. Let cool 5 minutes before slicing. Serve on a thick bed of spinach leaves and sprinkle generously with parsley.

Health Facilitators	Nutrient Density Rating
Protein	High
Fat	Moderate
Carbohydrate	High
Enzymes	High
Antioxidants	High
Fiber	High

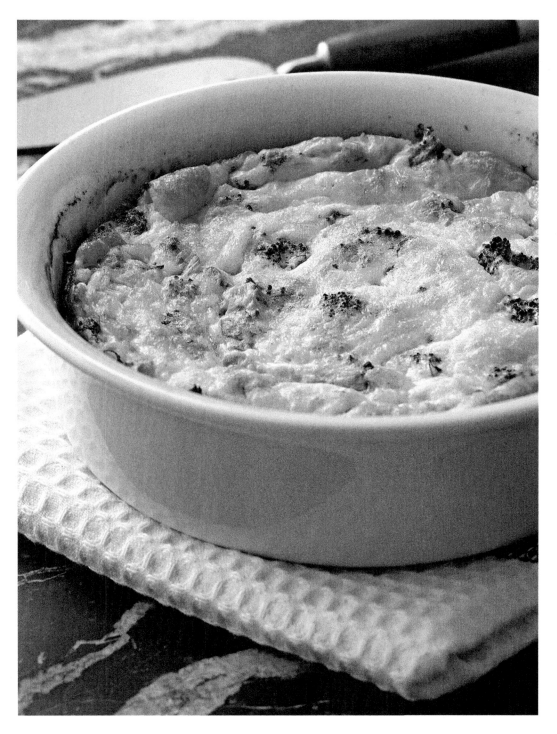

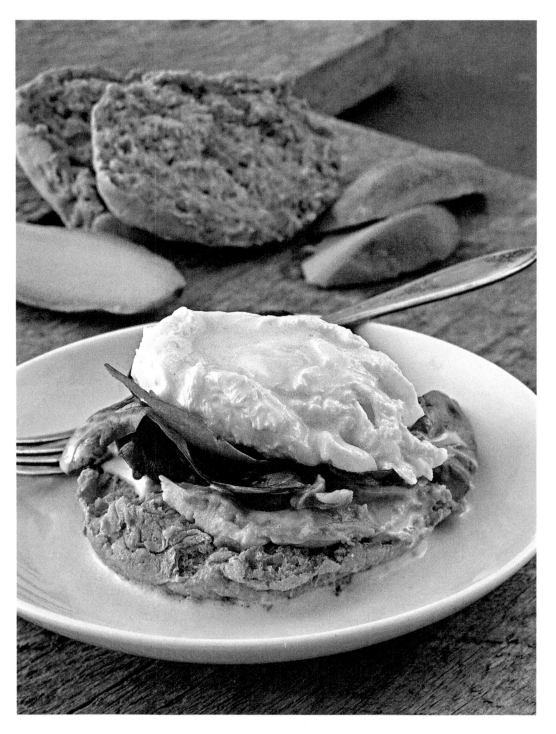

Eggs Florentine with Flair

Eggs are a great source of protein and vitamins A, D, and B, and spinach and avocado are loaded with extra enzymes and antioxidants. Add a healthy hollandaise sauce and whole-grain English muffins, and you turn this dish into a completely balanced and nourishing meal.

INGREDIENTS

For eggs

2 bunches fresh spinach leaves, washed
1 tablespoon (15 ml) apple cider vinegar
8 eggs
½ avocado, peeled and sliced
2 whole-grain English muffins sliced
 into halves or gluten-free bread

For hollandaise sauce

3 egg yolks
2 tablespoons (28 ml) fresh lemon juice
Dash cayenne pepper
4 ounces (112 g) unsalted butter, melted
 and bubbling hot

Yield: 4 servings

Health Facilitators	Nutrient Density Rating
Protein	High
Fat	Moderate
Carbohydrate	Moderate
Enzymes	Low
Antioxidants	High
Fiber	High

Place wet spinach (stems removed) into a steamer basket in a medium saucepan with a tight-fitting lid. Turn heat to medium-high and steam until leaves are wilted, about 2 to 3 minutes. Drain in a colander, pressing out all liquid. Chop and set aside.

In a large, deep skillet, bring 2 inches (5 cm) of water and vinegar to a boil over high heat. Reduce heat to a simmer. Crack eggs, one at a time, into a small bowl, then slide each egg gently into boiling water. Cover and cook 3 minutes for soft yolks, 5 minutes for firmer yolks. Using a slotted spoon, remove eggs from water.

To make sauce, in a blender, combine egg yolks, lemon juice, and cayenne pepper on high speed for 3 seconds. Remove the center section of the lid and, with motor running, slowly pour hot butter in a steady stream over eggs. Blend for an additional 5 seconds. Taste, and add more lemon juice or cayenne, if desired.

Toast the English muffins and spread with avocado slices. Arrange spinach on top of the muffin halves, followed by poached eggs. Top with warm hollandaise sauce.

Fisherman's Omega-3 Breakfast

Enjoy the delicious flavors of this wholesome trout or salmon and egg dish that's rich in omega-3 essential fatty acids. Paired with parsley and cilantro, which boast vitamin E, vitamin C, and many minerals, this dish is high in just about everything that's good for you—and it tastes great, too.

INGREDIENTS

1 teaspoon butter
Two 4-ounce (115-g) trout or salmon fillets
1 tablespoon (15 ml) apple cider vinegar
4 eggs
4 tablespoons (16 g) chopped fresh
  parsley
4 tablespoons (16 g) chopped fresh
  cilantro
4 to 6 romaine lettuce leaves
2 tablespoons (10 g) grated
  Parmesan cheese

Yield: 2 servings

Melt butter in a small bowl over hot water. Baste the trout or salmon with butter before lightly grilling over medium heat.

In a deep medium skillet, bring 2 inches (5 cm) of water and vinegar to a boil over high heat. Reduce heat to simmer. Crack an egg into a small bowl and tip gently into boiling water. Repeat with all eggs. Cover skillet and cook 3 minutes for soft yolks, 5 minutes for firmer yolks. Using a slotted spoon, remove the eggs from the water and drain thoroughly. Place each trout or salmon fillet on a bed of romaine lettuce and mixed parsley and cilantro. Top with two poached eggs and sprinkle with Parmesan cheese and more fresh parsley and cilantro. Serve immediately.

Health Facilitators	Nutrient Density Rating
Protein	High
Fat	Moderate
Carbohydrate	Moderate
Enzymes	High
Antioxidants	High
Fiber	High

DID YOU KNOW?

The role of fish in protecting against heart disease and cancer is well known, but there are many other benefits, such as decreasing inflammation and improving brain function.

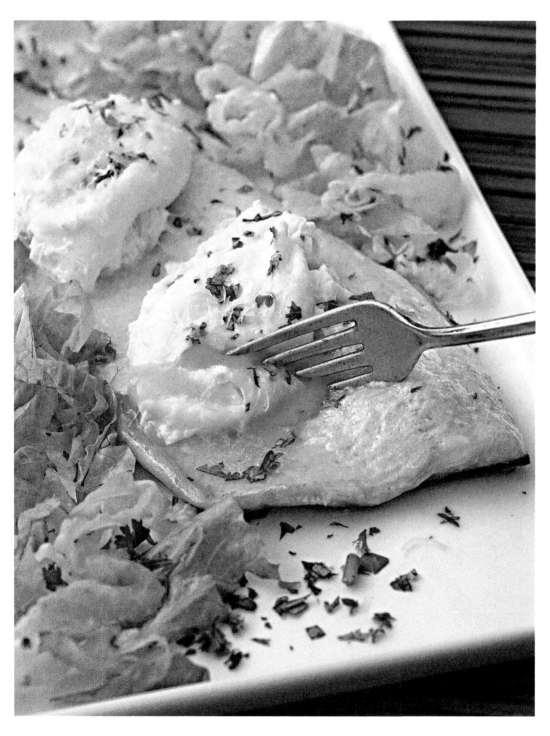

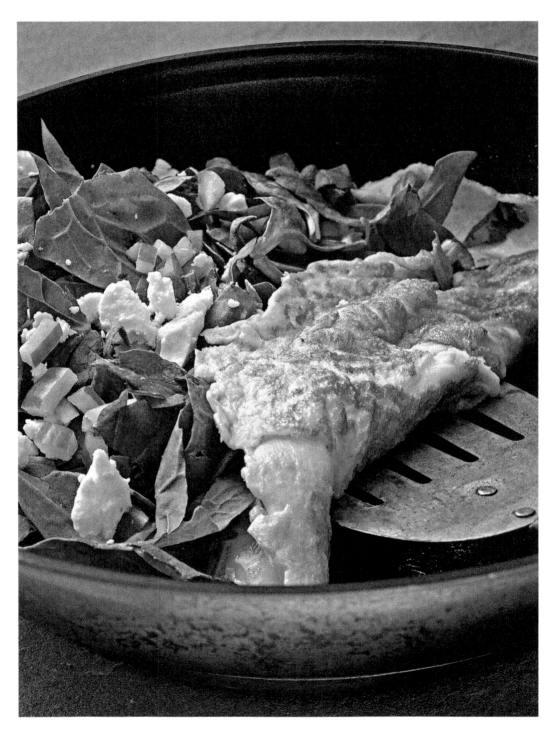

Popeye Prize Omelet

Stuff an already perfectly balanced omelet with Popeye's secret weapon—spinach. It's high in calcium, to build strong bones, as well as vitamins E and C. Garnish with plenty of salad greens and alfalfa sprouts for added enzymes, antioxidants, and fiber.

INGREDIENTS

For omelet

4 eggs

2 tablespoons (28 ml) heavy cream
    or yogurt

Freshly ground black pepper to taste

2 tablespoons (28 ml) olive oil

For filling

1 cup (225 g) cooked spinach,
    drained and chopped

3 tablespoons (28 g) crumbled
    goat cheese

2 tablespoons (5 g) finely slivered
    fresh basil, or 2 teaspoons dried basil

2 tablespoons (20 g) diced red onion

For garnish

1 slice whole grain rye or
    gluten-free bread

½ to 1 avocado, peeled and sliced

Salad greens and alfalfa sprouts

Yield: 2 servings

In a medium bowl, using a fork, whisk together eggs, cream, and black pepper. Set aside. Combine spinach with crumbled goat cheese, basil, and red onion. Set aside.

In a 10-inch (25-cm) skillet or frying pan, pour in 2 tablespoons (28 ml) olive oil. When the oil is hot, pour in the egg mixture. Cook over medium-high heat until eggs begin to set. Lift edges to allow uncooked egg to seep underneath.

When bottom layer of egg is cooked but top is still moist, spread spinach and cheese mixture over one side of omelet. Gently fold omelet in half. Cook half a minute longer until filling is hot.

Slide omelet onto a plate and serve immediately with plain or toasted rye bread spread with fresh avocado slices and garnished with salad greens and alfalfa sprouts.

Health Facilitators	Nutrient Density Rating
Protein	Very High
Fat	Moderate
Carbohydrate	Moderate
Enzymes	Moderate
Antioxidants	Low
Fiber	High

Sunshine Cheese and Herb Soufflés

Benefits abound in the wide array of vitamins, minerals, fats, and proteins from the eggs and dairy products in this delicious dish. The herbs are strong in phytonutrients and anti-oxidants for added vitamins and minerals.

INGREDIENTS

4 tablespoons (55 g) butter, plus
  1 teaspoon for greasing ramekins
1/3 cup (40 g) gluten-free flour
2 cups (470 ml) milk
1 cup (120 g) grated aged cheddar
  cheese
6 eggs, separated
4 tablespoons (16 g) chopped fresh dill,
  divided
2 tablespoons (5 g) chopped fresh basil
2 tablespoons (8 g) chopped fresh
  cilantro
3 tablespoons (15 g) grated Parmesan
  cheese
Salt and freshly ground black pepper

Yield: 6 servings

Health Facilitators	Nutrient Density Rating
Protein	Very High
Fat	High
Carbohydrate	Moderate
Enzymes	Moderate
Antioxidants	High
Fiber	Low

Preheat oven to 400°F (200°C, or gas mark 6). In a large saucepan, melt the butter and add the flour. Cook for 2 minutes, stirring continuously, and then gradually add the milk, stirring. Simmer until thickened, then allow to cool. Stir the cheddar cheese, egg yolks, 3 tablespoons (12 g) dill, basil, and cilantro into the sauce. Beat the egg whites with a pinch of salt until stiff. Stir one quarter of the egg whites into the cheese sauce, then fold in the remainder.

Butter six small ramekins and dust with Parmesan cheese. Divide the mixture among the ramekins. Bake for 15-20 minutes, until the soufflés are puffed and golden brown. Garnish with the remaining table-spoon (4 g) chopped dill, and serve immediately.

Did You Know?

The latest research now recognizes the many health benefits of eggs, which include preventing circulatory problems, such as clotting, heart disease, and stroke, as well as promoting healthy neurotransmitter function for sending messages between nerves and muscles.

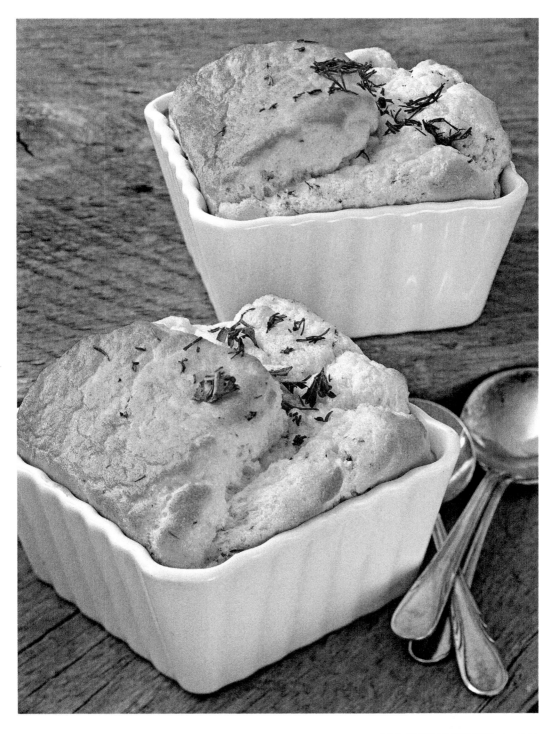

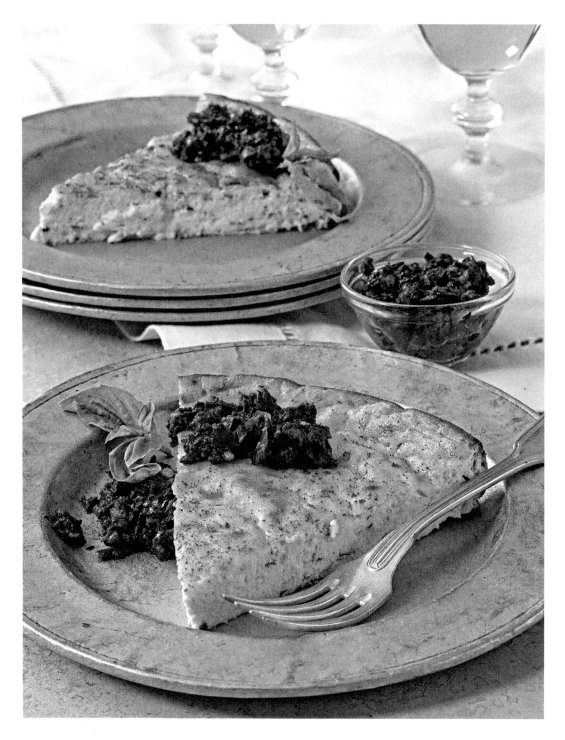

Italian Herb and Ricotta Cheese Flan

Calcium-rich ricotta cheese forms the basis of this immune-boosting dish. Garlic is Mother Nature's secret weapon to boost the immune system and reduce inflammation. With its antibacterial, antiviral, and anti-fungal activity, it works against intestinal parasites and has yielded long-term success with recurrent yeast infections. Combined with the fresh herbs, tapenade, and Parmesan cheese, this dish is a medicinal delight.

INGREDIENTS

For flan

Olive oil, for greasing and glazing
3½ cups (875 g) ricotta cheese
1 cup (100 g) grated Parmesan cheese
3 eggs, separated
4 tablespoons (10 g) torn fresh basil
   leaves, plus four whole leaves for garnish
5 tablespoons (15 g) fresh chives, divided
4 tablespoons (16 g) fresh oregano
   leaves, divided
½ teaspoon salt
Freshly ground black pepper
½ teaspoon paprika

For tapenade

3½ cups (350 g) pitted black olives,
   halved
5 garlic cloves, peeled and crushed
5 tablespoons (75 ml) pure-pressed olive oil

Yield: 6 servings

Preheat oven to 350°F (180°C, or gas mark 4) and lightly oil a 9-inch (23-cm) spring-form cake pan. Mix together the ricotta cheese, Parmesan cheese, and egg yolks in a food processor. Add torn basil leaves, 4 tablespoons (12 g) chives, 3 tablespoons (12 g) oregano, salt, pepper, and paprika, and blend until smooth.

Whisk egg whites in a large bowl until they form soft peaks, and then gently fold into the ricotta mixture. Spoon into the cake pan and smooth over the top.

Bake for 1 hour 20 minutes or until the flan has risen and the top is golden. Remove from the oven, brush lightly with olive oil, and sprinkle with paprika. Leave to cool before removing from the cake pan.

For the tapenade, process the olive halves and garlic in a food processor until finely chopped. Gradually add the olive oil and blend to a coarse paste, then transfer to a serving bowl.

Garnish the flan with whole basil leaves and remaining chives and oregano, and serve with tapenade.

Health Facilitators	Nutrient Density Rating
Protein	High
Fat	High
Carbohydrate	Moderate
Enzymes	Moderate
Antioxidants	Low
Fiber	Low

Lean and Light Tofu Scrambler

This scramble is a well-balanced breakfast that's also delicious as a light lunch or dinner. The eggs and tofu are excellent sources of protein and healthy fat. By serving it with parsley, peppers, avocado, and romaine lettuce, the dish provides an abundance of anti-inflammatory vegetables that are also high in fiber, enzymes, and antioxidants.

INGREDIENTS
1 large egg
1 tablespoon (15 ml) rice or soy milk
Salt and pepper to taste
¼ cup (40 g) chopped onion
¼ cup (30 g) chopped green pepper
1 teaspoon olive oil
3 ounces (85 g) tofu
2 large romaine leaves
1 slice rye or pumpernickel bread
¼ fresh avocado, peeled and mashed
⅓ cup (20 g) fresh chopped parsley

Yield: 1 serving

Health Facilitators	Nutrient Density Rating
Protein	High
Fat	Moderate
Carbohydrate	Moderate
Enzymes	Moderate
Antioxidants	Moderate
Fiber	Moderate

Combine egg, milk, salt, and pepper in a bowl and beat slightly. In a frying pan, sauté the onion and green pepper in olive oil until tender. Crumble tofu into the pan. Add egg mixture and cook until firm. Serve immediately on a bed of romaine lettuce and bread spread generously with fresh avocado. Sprinkle with fresh parsley.

Did You Know?
Tofu is rich in soy isoflavones, genistein, and daidzein, which are phytonutrients. Firm tofu contains about 35 mg isoflavones per 100 g. Isoflavones have been known to reduce the risk of osteoporosis, lower rates of breast cancer and prostate cancer, and reduce menopausal symptoms including mood swings and hot flushes.

Tofu also reduces the risk of heart disease by lowering high blood pressure and the level of the "bad" LDL cholesterol in the blood.

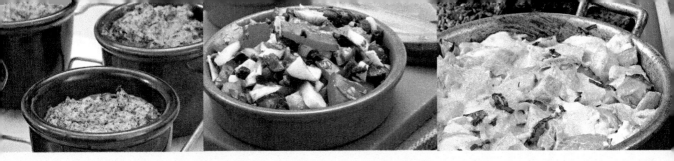

HEALTHY SNACKING

Powerful Pumpkin Seed Dip (RAW)

Pumpkin seeds are high in zinc, a powerful immune-system booster. They are also high in iron, calcium, magnesium, copper, vitamin E, and essential fatty acids for added inflammatory benefits. They are a good source of protein and contain a nice balance of amino acids, including tryptophan. Toss in some lemon or lime juice, parsley, and herbs, and it becomes super-charged.

INGREDIENTS

2 cups (280 g) pumpkin seeds, soaked in purified or spring water overnight and drained

½ cup (28 g) sun-dried tomatoes, soaked in purified or spring water overnight and drained

1 tablespoon (4 g) fresh parsley, finely minced

1 tablespoon (4 g) fresh oregano, finely minced

1 tablespoon (2.5 g) fresh thyme, finely minced

2 tablespoons (28 ml) pure-pressed extra-virgin olive oil

1 tablespoon (15 ml) lemon juice

1 teaspoon Himalayan crystal salt

Yield: 2½ cups (590 ml)

Process pumpkin seeds and sun-dried tomatoes in a food processor until they are smooth and creamy. Add fresh herbs along with other ingredients. Mix well, and serve with freshly cut vegetables and/or flax crackers. The dip will last for a few days in the refrigerator.

Did You Know?

Pumpkin seeds, also known as pepitas, are high in carotenoids, omega-3 fats, and zinc. The carotenoids and the omega-3 fats found in the seeds are being studied for their potential benefits to the prostate gland. Studies have shown that men with higher amounts of carotenoids in their diet have less risk for benign prostatic hypertrophy, or BPH.

Health Facilitators	Nutrient Density Rating
Protein	Very High
Fat	High
Carbohydrate	High
Enzymes	Very High
Antioxidants	Very High
Fiber	High

Brain Food Walnut Dip (RAW)

Walnuts are a good source of all-important omega-3 fatty acids, and they provide health benefits ranging from cardiovascular protection and improved mental function to anti-inflammatory help with asthma, rheumatoid arthritis, eczema, and psoriasis.

INGREDIENTS
2 cups (200 g) walnuts, shelled
1 cup (90 g) leeks, finely chopped
2 tablespoons (28 ml) pure-pressed extra-virgin olive oil
1 teaspoon each of dried or fresh oregano, parsley, thyme, and basil
1 teaspoon Himalayan crystal salt

Yield: 2½ cups (590 ml)

Process all ingredients in a food processor until smooth and creamy, adding a little water for consistency. Serve with flax crackers or freshly cut vegetables, such as carrots and celery.

Did You Know?

In addition to its many health benefits, walnuts contain an antioxidant compound called ellagic acid that supports the immune system and appears to have several anti-cancer properties. Walnuts have also been shown to aid in the lowering of "bad" LDL cholesterol and the C-reactive protein (CRP), which was recently recognized as being an independent marker and predictor of heart disease.

Health Facilitators	Nutrient Density Rating
Protein	Very High
Fat	Very High
Carbohydrate	Moderate
Enzymes	High
Antioxidants	Moderate
Fiber	High

Mediterranean Cheese and Herb Dip (RAW)

This Mediterranean-style dip is packed with antioxidants and phytonutrients. The variety of herbs, together with the creamy texture of avocado and Gorgonzola cheese, will delight your taste buds, while providing immune system benefits. This dip is wonderful as an accompaniment to crackers, pears, apples, peaches, nuts, or raisins or made into a sauce for chicken.

INGREDIENTS

2 large ripe avocados
½ cup (60 g) crumbled Gorgonzola cheese
1 cup (230 g) whole-milk sour cream
1 tablespoon (14 g) mayonnaise
2 tablespoons (28 ml) fresh lime juice
3 tablespoons (18 g) chopped scallions
3 tablespoons (12 g) chopped fresh cilantro
3 tablespoons (12 g) chopped Italian parsley
2 garlic cloves, minced
Dash cayenne pepper
Freshly ground black pepper to taste

Yield: 2½ cups (590 ml)

Cut avocados in half. Remove pits, scoop flesh into a medium bowl, and mash coarsely with a fork. Add Gorgonzola cheese, sour cream, and mayonnaise, and blend well. Add lime juice, scallions, cilantro, parsley, garlic, cayenne, and black pepper. Blend until well mixed. Taste, and adjust seasonings. Chill 1 hour before serving. Serve in a medium bowl with cut-up raw vegetables and/or flax crackers.

Did You Know?

Avocados contain potassium, folate, and monosaturated fats, and are very high in fiber. The monosaturated fats in avocados contain oleic acid, which has been found to improve fat levels in the body and help control diabetes by lowering triglycerides.

Health Facilitators	Nutrient Density Rating
Protein	High
Fat	High
Carbohydrate	Moderate
Enzymes	High
Antioxidants	High
Fiber	High

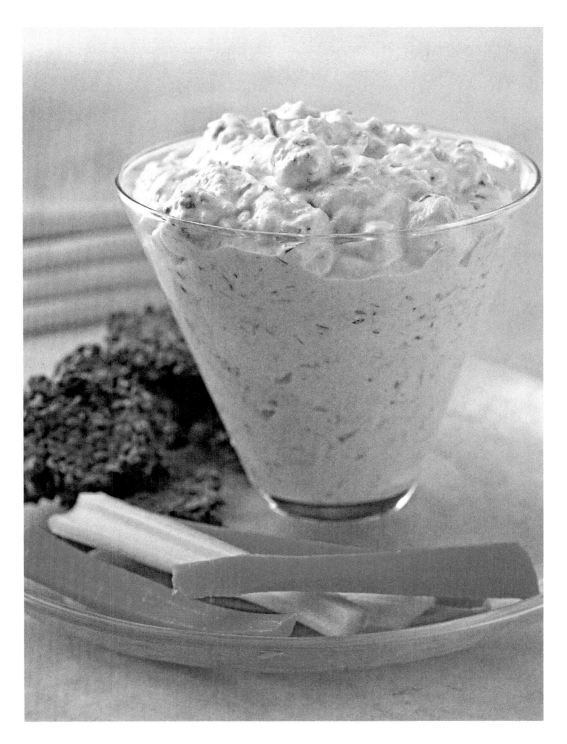

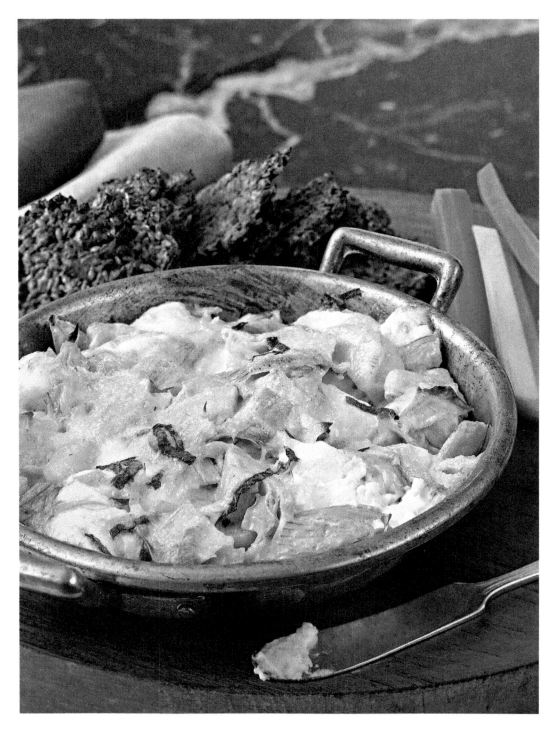

Hot Italian Artichoke Dip

Enjoy this delicious Italian delicacy. Artichokes are rich in fiber, folic acid, and potassium. Antioxidants such as vitamins A and C combine with calcium and magnesium to make this dip nutritious and beneficial.

INGREDIENTS

13¾-ounce (425 ml) can or jar of artichoke hearts in water, drained and rinsed
8 ounces (225 g) cream cheese, diced into small cubes
$^1/_3$ cup (75 g) mayonnaise
$^2/_3$ cup (65 g) grated Parmesan cheese
2 tablespoons (5 g) slivered fresh basil
1 teaspoon grated lemon zest
Freshly ground black pepper to taste
Dash cayenne pepper

Yield: 3 cups (710 ml)

Preheat oven to 425°F (220°C, or gas mark 7). Coarsely chop drained artichoke hearts. Mix with cream cheese, mayonnaise, Parmesan cheese, basil, lemon zest, black pepper, and cayenne pepper. Transfer to a lightly oiled ovenproof casserole dish or 9-inch (23 cm) pie pan and bake for 20 minutes, or until dip is bubbling hot. Serve with cut-up raw vegetables and/or flax crackers.

Health Facilitators	Nutrient Density Rating
Protein	Moderate
Fat	High
Carbohydrate	High
Enzymes	High
Antioxidants	High
Fiber	High

Nutrient-Dense Hummus

The spread contains spinach—high in iron, calcium, and vitamin A—plus it has fiber, antioxidants, and protein. It gets a hit of vitamin B from garbanzo beans and plenty of protein, zinc, copper, magnesium, vitamin E, and additional calcium from the tahini. Garlic gives a good boost to your immune system. Hummus is great spread over raw flax crackers or fresh, sliced raw vegetables.

INGREDIENTS

2 cups (500 g) dried garbanzo beans
3 cloves garlic, finely chopped
1 cup (180 g) cooked spinach, well drained and chopped
½ cup (120 ml) fresh lemon juice
½ cup (120 g) sesame tahini
¼ cup (60 ml) pure-pressed extra-virgin olive oil
½ teaspoon ground cumin
Dash of cayenne pepper
1 tablespoon (15 ml) flaxseed oil
Dash of paprika (optional)

Yield: 2½ to 3 cups (595 to 610 ml)

Soak garbanzo beans in purified water overnight. Drain and place them in a saucepan with enough fresh water to cover. Cook gently for 20 to 30 minutes, remove from heat, and drain.

In a food processor, combine drained beans with garlic, spinach, lemon juice, sesame tahini, olive oil, cumin, cayenne pepper, and flaxseed oil until well blended. Taste, and adjust seasonings, adding more lemon juice if desired. Place dip in a medium serving bowl, sprinkle with paprika, if desired, and serve.

Health Facilitators	Nutrient Density Rating
Protein	High
Fat	Moderate
Carbohydrate	High
Enzymes	High
Antioxidants	High
Fiber	High

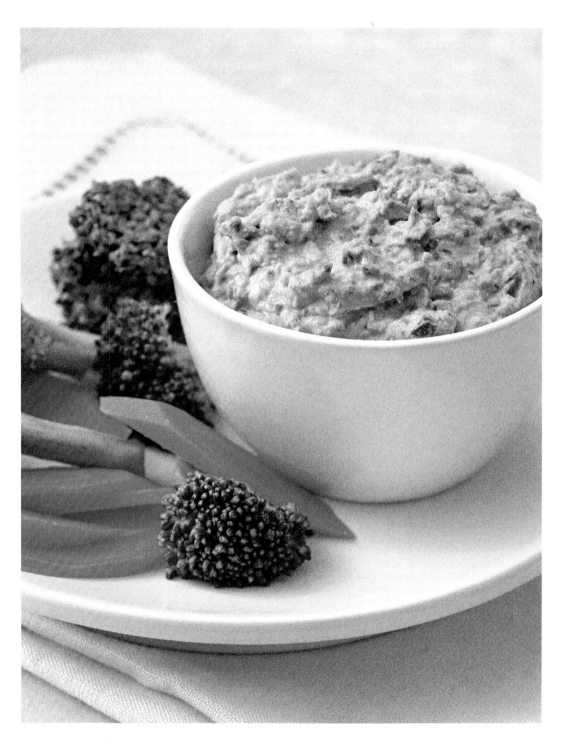

Lemon Tahini (RAW)

Nourish yourself with lemon tahini made from sesame seeds, which contain protein (20 percent) vitamins A and E, and most of the B vitamins except B12 and folic acid. Minerals are even more abundant in sesame seeds, particularly zinc, calcium, copper, magnesium, phosphorus, and potassium.

INGREDIENTS

2 cups (290 g) white sesame seeds, soaked overnight in purified water and drained
1 cup (235 ml) purified water
½ cup (120 ml) lemon juice
1 teaspoon Himalayan crystal salt

Yield: 2 cups (475 ml)

In a blender, process all ingredients until smooth and creamy. Refrigerate and serve with freshly cut vegetables or flax crackers.

Did You Know?

Sesame seeds are an excellent source of calcium. They also have a mild antioxidant effect, possibly because of their vitamin E content.

Health Facilitators	Nutrient Density Rating
Protein	High
Fat	High
Carbohydrate	Moderate
Enzymes	High
Antioxidants	High
Fiber	High

Spring Salsa (RAW)

Get a fresh start with this antioxidant-rich, vitamin-packed tangy salsa. The green and red peppers are high in vitamin C, bioflavonoids, and vitamin A, which are all antioxidants that keep the immune system healthy. Your immune system will love the additional antioxidant benefits from the garlic and lemon juice.

INGREDIENTS

7 ripe tomatoes, diced
½ cup (30 g) fresh cilantro, finely chopped
½ cup (30 g) fresh parsley, finely chopped
1 green pepper, finely chopped
1 red pepper, finely chopped
1 yellow onion, finely chopped
6 cloves garlic, minced
2 tablespoons (6 g) fresh chives, finely chopped
2 tablespoons (28 ml) lemon juice
2 tablespoons (28 ml) lime juice
1 tablespoon (15 ml) apple cider vinegar
Cumin to taste
1 teaspoon cayenne pepper
Dash salt

Yield: 6 to 8 cups (1350 to 1800 g)

Combine all ingredients in a mixing bowl and serve with freshly cut vegetables and/or flax crackers.

Did You Know?
Whole tomatoes contain some vitamin E, folic acid, and other B vitamins, such as biotin and niacin, and a bit of iron, sodium, calcium, magnesium, and zinc, in addition to an abundance of lycopene.

Health Facilitators	Nutrient Density Rating
Protein	Low
Fat	Low
Carbohydrate	High
Enzymes	High
Antioxidants	High
Fiber	High

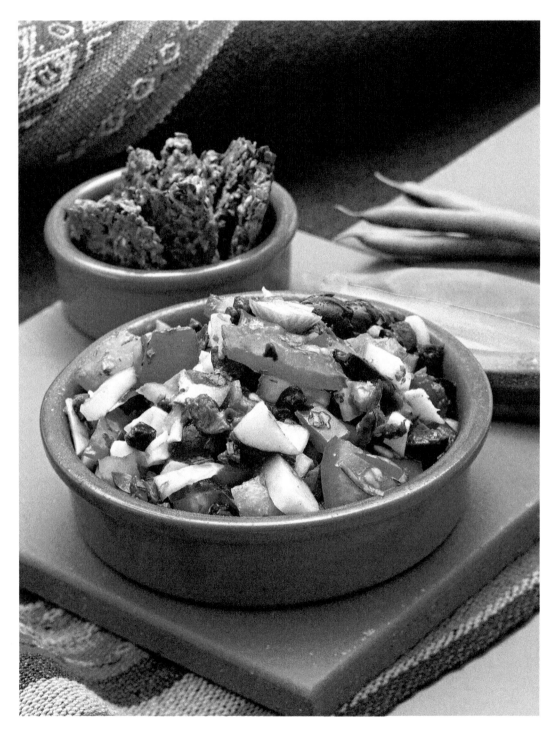

Spanish Olé Salsa (RAW)

Fresh and canned tomatoes contain the antioxidant lycopene, which enhances the functioning of our immune system by boosting production and maintenance of our natural killer cells—also referred to as white blood cells. White blood cells are quite powerful—they are capable of destroying more than 100 types of viruses and bacteria, and many different types of cancer cells.

INGREDIENTS

3 tomatoes, chopped
1 cucumber, chopped
1 cup (100 g) black olives, pitted and
  chopped
½ cup (45 g) fresh fennel, chopped
½ cup (30 g) fresh cilantro, chopped
2 teaspoons cayenne pepper
2 teaspoons cumin
1 teaspoon lime juice
1 teaspoon Himalayan crystal salt

Yield: 2½ cups (680 ml)

Stir all ingredients together by hand. Chill and serve with freshly cut vegetables or flax crackers.

Did You Know?

Olives are a delicious source of antioxidants and phytonutrients, namely polyphenols. Polyphenols give olives their taste and aroma and are thought to have anti-inflammatory properties.

Health Facilitators	Nutrient Density Rating
Protein	Moderate
Fat	High
Carbohydrate	High
Enzymes	High
Antioxidants	High
Fiber	High

Get-Up-and-Go Chutney (RAW)

This apricot-raisin chutney will give you vim and vitality. Apricots have health-building virtues. Whether fresh or dried, this fruit is rich in easily digestible natural sugars, vitamins A and C, riboflavin (B2), and niacin (B3). Raisins provide a healthy dose of iron, potassium, calcium, and magnesium, all of which are great for energy pick-up.

INGREDIENTS
½ cup (75 g) raisins
½ cup (65 g) dried apricots
½ cup (120 ml) boiling water
2 tablespoons (28 ml) fresh lime juice
Dash cayenne pepper

Yield: 1 cup (235 ml)

In a small bowl, soak raisins and apricots in boiling water for 15 minutes. Transfer to a blender or food processor and add lime juice and cayenne pepper. Process until well blended and smooth. Taste, and adjust seasonings. Cover and refrigerate. Serve on crackers or with Indian curries.

Did You Know?
Apricots are also an excellent source of minerals such as calcium, phosphorus, and iron, and deliver traces of sodium, sulphur, manganese, cobalt, and bromine.

Health Facilitators	Nutrient Density Rating
Protein	Low
Fat	Low
Carbohydrate	High
Enzymes	High
Antioxidants	High
Fiber	High

Digestive Goat Cheese with Pistachio Nuts Spread (RAW)

Most lactose intolerants who can't have cow's milk are able to digest goat's milk. To increase the benefits of this dip, make it without the cream cheese and double the amount of goat cheese, which also happens to be higher in enzymes than cow's cheese.

INGREDIENTS

3 ounces (85 g) chevre (goat cheese)
3 ounces (85 g) cream cheese, softened to room temperature
1 tablespoon (15 ml) all-dairy heavy cream
$1/3$ cup (40 g) finely chopped dry-roasted pistachio nuts, plus ¼ cup (35 g) chopped dry-roasted pistachio nuts for garnish
Dash cayenne pepper
$1/3$ cup (20 g) chopped parsley

Yield: 1 cup (235 ml)

In a medium bowl, using a fork, blend chevre, cream cheese, cream, chopped pistachio nuts, and cayenne pepper. Transfer to a serving bowl and top with reserved pistachio nuts. Serve with flax crackers or spread on apple and pear slices or celery sticks.

Did You Know?

Pistachios are wonderful sources of potassium, iron, and magnesium, plus other trace minerals for balancing the digestive system.

Health Facilitators	Nutrient Density Rating
Protein	High
Fat	Moderate
Carbohydrate	High
Enzymes	Moderate
Antioxidants	Moderate
Fiber	Moderate

Almighty Almond Butter Spread (RAW)

Almonds are low in saturated fat and contain many other protective nutrients, including calcium and magnesium (for strong bones), vitamin E, and phytochemicals. Almonds also have been shown to help protect against cardiovascular disease and even cancer. If you'd prefer a different nut, you can substitute peanuts or cashews for the almonds.

INGREDIENTS

2 cups (290 g) raw almonds, soaked in
  purified water overnight and drained
1 teaspoon Himalayan crystal salt
2 tablespoons (40 g) raw honey
¾ cup (175 ml) coconut oil

Yield: 2 cups (475 ml)

Health Facilitators	Nutrient Density Rating
Protein	High
Fat	Very High
Carbohydrate	Moderate
Enzymes	High
Antioxidants	Low
Fiber	High

Place nuts and salt in food processor and grind to a fine powder. Add honey and coconut oil and process until mixture becomes smooth, like butter. It will be somewhat liquid but will harden when chilled. Store in an airtight container in the refrigerator. Serve at room temperature with flax crackers or freshly cut vegetables, such as carrot and celery.

Did You Know?

New research gives even more support to the healthy benefits of almonds: almonds may help fight obesity and diabetes. This is partly because almonds help slow the actual absorption of carbohydrates into the body, which means that they help to create a slower rise in blood sugar levels, thereby keeping insulin levels in check.

Peanut Butter Apple Mint Spread (RAW)

Peanuts are high in protein and healthy fat. Apples are high in fiber, and apple pectin has a detoxifying quality that is used in many cleansing formulas. Combine these two delicious ingredients together with some fresh mint and you'll discover a delightful taste sensation.

INGREDIENTS

1 cup (150 g) apple, peeled, cored, and chopped
¼ cup (65 g) peanut butter (no sugar added)
1 teaspoon fresh chopped mint leaves

Yield: 1 cup (235 ml)

Purée the apple in a blender. Place apple purée and peanut butter together in a bowl and blend until smooth. Add the mint and refrigerate. Spread over flax crackers, or serve with freshly cut vegetables, such as carrot and celery.

Did You Know?

The versatile peanut is an excellent source of thiamin, niacin, potassium, and magnesium, and a good source of pantothenic acid, zinc, and phosphorus, all of which support healthy immune function. There's even a little bit of iron thrown in for good nutritional measure.

Health Facilitators	Nutrient Density Rating
Protein	High
Fat	High
Carbohydrate	High
Enzymes	High
Antioxidants	High
Fiber	High

Italian Sun-Dried Tomato Flax Crackers

The benefits of flaxseeds are numerous—they improve the flow of every system in the body and have a gentle laxative action. Flaxseeds are high in omega-3 oils, which the body needs daily and does not produce on its own. These crunchy flax crackers are a healthy accompaniment to soups, salads, or any of the dip recipes in this book.

INGREDIENTS
1 bunch fresh parsley
2 cups (110 g) sun-dried tomatoes (dry-packed not oil-packed), soaked in spring water overnight, and drained
4 cups (675 g) flaxseeds, soaked in purified water for 10 to 20 minutes and drained
2 tablespoons (6 g) dried Italian seasoning
1 tablespoon (15 ml) olive oil
1 teaspoon Himalayan crystal salt
1 teaspoon cayenne pepper

Yield: 80 to 100 crackers

Blend sun-dried tomatoes and parsley in a processor until smooth. Scrape tomatoes and parsley into a large mixing bowl, add the soaked flaxseeds and all remaining ingredients, and mix well. Using a trowel or spatula, spread mixture approximately $1/8$ inch (3 mm) thick on dehydrator trays with a Teflex sheet. Dehydrate at 145°F (63°C) for 2 to 3 hours, then turn over, remove Teflex, and continue dehydrating for 6 to 8 hours at 115°F (46°C), or until desired crispness is reached. Store in glass containers.

Did You Know?
Sun-dried tomatoes are high in vitamin C and lycopene, two well-known antioxidants that help fight inflammation.

Health Facilitators	Nutrient Density Rating
Protein	High
Fat	High
Carbohydrate	High
Enzymes	High
Antioxidants	High
Fiber	High

Kale Curry Crackers

Kale is rich in calcium, iron, and vitamins A, C, and K. Moreover, these crackers are high in fiber and antioxidants such as vitamin E. The addition of curry powder will delight your taste buds while promoting numerous health benefits, such as purifying the blood, strengthening digestion, and improving intestinal flora. Curry powder also aids in the digestion of protein and helps relieve congestion.

INGREDIENTS

1 cup (145 g) almonds, soaked overnight, then drained
1 cup (70 g) kale
2 cups (225 g) flaxseeds, ground
1 tablespoon (6 g) curry powder
1 teaspoon ground cumin
1 teaspoon Himalayan crystal salt

Yield: Approximately 40 crackers

Process almonds and kale through a juicer or in a food processor. Add to remaining ingredients in large bowl and mix well. Using a trowel or a spatula, spread mixture approximately $1/8$ inch (3 mm) thick on dehydrator trays with a Teflex sheet. Dehydrate at 145°F (63°C) for 2 to 3 hours, then turn over, remove Teflex, and continue dehydrating for 6 to 8 hours at 115°F (46°C), or until desired crispness is reached. Store in glass containers.

Did You Know?

Kale has seven times the beta-carotene of broccoli and ten times more lutein.

Health Facilitators	Nutrient Density Rating
Protein	High
Fat	High
Carbohydrate	High
Enzymes	High
Antioxidants	High
Fiber	High

Turkey Avocado Roll-Ups

Relax and feel nourished with this delicious treat that's as easy to make as it is slimming for the waistline. Turkey is high in tryptophan, a feel-good neurochemical that calms your mood. The addition of healthy fats from avocado and heart-healthy cayenne pepper makes this an anytime pick-me-up snack. Great at bedtime, too.

INGREDIENTS
½ avocado, mashed or sliced
6 slices low-sodium, nitrate-free, oven-baked turkey
Dash of cayenne pepper (optional)
1 cup (55 g) chopped romaine lettuce

Yield: 6 roll-ups

Spread the avocado over each slice of turkey and roll up. Add a dash of cayenne pepper. Serve with a sprinkle of the romaine lettuce.

Health Facilitators	Nutrient Density Rating
Protein	High
Fat	Low
Carbohydrate	Low
Enzymes	High
Antioxidants	High
Fiber	Moderate

Crispy Nuts

In a nutshell, nuts are high in protein and fiber and very high in the minerals magnesium and potassium. Shaped like a mini-sized brain, walnuts are also brain food. They are high in omega-3 fatty acids, too, so you can say goodbye to brain fog.

INGREDIENTS

4 cups (580 g) raw, unsalted walnuts, almonds, pecans, and/or Brazil nuts
1 teaspoon sea salt or Himalayan salt
2 cups (470 ml) filtered water

Yield: 4 cups (400 g)

Place the nuts in a bowl with the salt and cover with the filtered water. Cover the bowl and allow the nuts to soak at room temperature overnight. Preheat the oven to 150°F (66°C). Drain the nuts in a colander and scatter onto a baking tray or cookie sheet. Place in the oven for up to 6 hours, or until completely dry and crisp. Store in an airtight container in a cool place or refrigerate. Add raisins, dried fruits, or sunflower seeds as you wish.

Health Facilitators	Nutrient Density Rating
Protein	High
Fat	Moderate
Carbohydrate	Low
Enzymes	High
Antioxidants	High
Fiber	High

Cleansing Thai Tempeh Cakes

Many of the ingredients in this dish are excellent sources of vitamins A, B, C, and E, plus minerals such as potassium and folate. The chilies and cilantro act as detoxifiers t hat remove waste products from our body and increase the supply of nutrients to tissues. They stimulate the release of endorphins, which are natural pain killers and are effective in relieving rheumatoid arthritis and osteoarthritis.

INGREDIENTS

1 lemon grass stalk, outer leaves removed and inside finely chopped
2 garlic cloves, chopped
2 scallions, finely chopped
2 chili peppers, seeded and finely chopped (any variety you prefer)
1-inch (2.5-cm) piece fresh ginger root, peeled and finely chopped
4 tablespoons (16 g) chopped fresh cilantro plus 1 tablespoon (4 g) for garnish
2¼ cups (375 g) tempeh, defrosted if frozen, sliced
1 tablespoon (15 ml) lime juice
1 teaspoon brown sugar
3 tablespoons (24 g) whole wheat or gluten-free flour
1 large egg, lightly beaten
Dash of Himalayan crystal salt and freshly ground black pepper
2 to 3 tablespoons (20 to 26 ml) olive oil

Yield: 8 servings

Place the lemon grass, garlic, scallions, chili peppers, ginger, and cilantro in a food processor or blender and process to a coarse paste. Add tempeh, lime juice, and brown sugar and blend until combined. Add the flour, egg, and salt and pepper to taste. Process again until mixture forms a coarse, sticky paste.

Divide the tempeh mixture into 8 equal parts. Form into balls with your hands. The mixture will be quite sticky, so it may help to flour your hands at intervals.

Press the balls flat to form small cakes about ¾ inch (2 cm) thick.

Heat olive oil in large frying pan. Fry tempeh cakes for 5 to 6 minutes, turning once, until golden. Drain cakes on paper towel and serve warm with dipping sauce (recipe on page 138), garnished with chopped cilantro.

Health Facilitators	Nutrient Density Rating
Protein	High
Fat	Low
Carbohydrate	High
Enzymes	Moderate
Antioxidants	Very High
Fiber	High

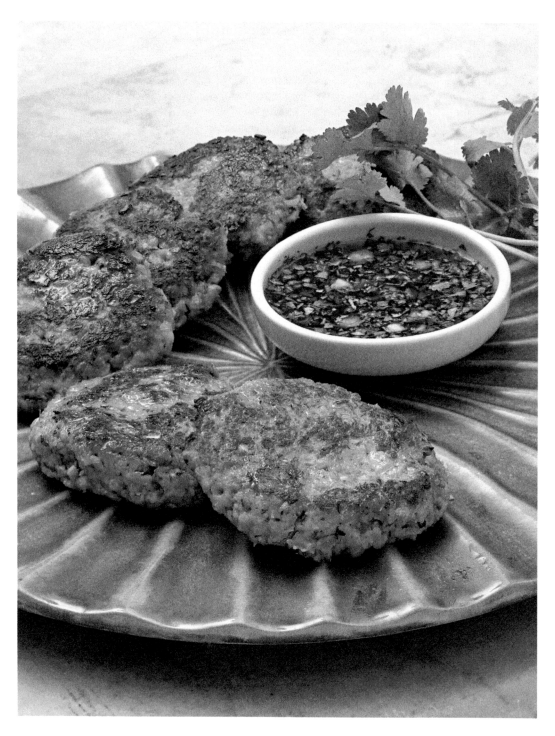

Sweet Dipping Sauce

INGREDIENTS
3 tablespoons (45 ml) mirin
3 tablespoons (45 ml) white wine vinegar
2 scallions, finely sliced
1 tablespoon (15 g) brown sugar
2 chili peppers, finely chopped
2 tablespoons (8 g) chopped fresh
  cilantro
Large pinch Himalayan crystal salt

Mix together the mirin, white wine vinegar, sliced scallions, sugar, chili peppers, chopped fresh cilantro, and salt in a small bowl. Serve with Thai tempeh cakes.

Did You Know?
Mirin, a low-alcohol, sweet wine made from glutinous rice, is an essential ingredient for Japanese cooking. It can be found in the Asian section of most supermarkets.

Crispy Nuts

In a nutshell, nuts are high in protein and fiber, and very high in fat-healthy fat.

INGREDIENTS
4 cups (580 g) raw nuts: pecans, walnuts, almonds (whole skinless, slivered or sliced), macadamias, peanuts, or cashews
1 tablespoon (18 g) Himalayan crystal salt
Pure water

Yield: 4 cups (580 g)

Place nuts in a bowl with salt and cover with water. Cover bowl loosely and leave at room temperature for about 8 hours. (Note: Soak cashews for up to 6 hours.) Drain in a colander and scatter on a stainless steel baking pan or cookie sheet. Place in oven set at 150°F (65°C) (or lower) and dehydrate for 12 to 24 hours or until completely dry and crisp. You can also use a food dehydrator. Store in an air-tight container in a cool place or refrigerate.

Did You Know?
Soaking nuts overnight and then lightly roasting them at a low temperature in the oven for several hours on (or placing them in a food dehydrator) not only brings out their flavor but also improves their digestibility, because the enzyme-inhibitors are released, providing you with all their nutrients.

Health Facilitators	Nutrient Density Rating
Protein	High
Fat	Very High
Carbohydrate	Low
Enzymes	High
Antioxidants	Low
Fiber	High

Antiox-Artichokes with Hollandaise Sauce

Mother Nature outdid herself with the artichoke's beautiful packaging and exquisite taste. Artichokes are loaded with potassium, which is vital for supporting muscle and nerve function; magnesium, which is used for building strong bones and for releasing energy from muscle storage; and vitamin C, a potent antioxidant. Moreover, they are fiber-rich, helping to maintain a healthy digestive system and to keep blood-sugar levels stable.

INGREDIENTS
4 fresh artichokes
1 lemon, cut in quarters
Hollandaise sauce (page 105)

Yield: 4 servings

With a sharp knife, slice the top from each artichoke and trim the stems, so that they sit upright. Use kitchen shears to trim points off the ends of the leaves. Place artichokes, along with a quartered lemon, in 4 inches (10 cm) of boiling water. Boil uncovered about 35 to 45 minutes, or until leaves are tender and pull away easily.

Serve with hollandaise sauce on the side, in dipping bowls.

Health Facilitators	Nutrient Density Rating
Protein	High
Fat	Moderate
Carbohydrate	High
Enzymes	High
Antioxidants	High
Fiber	Very High

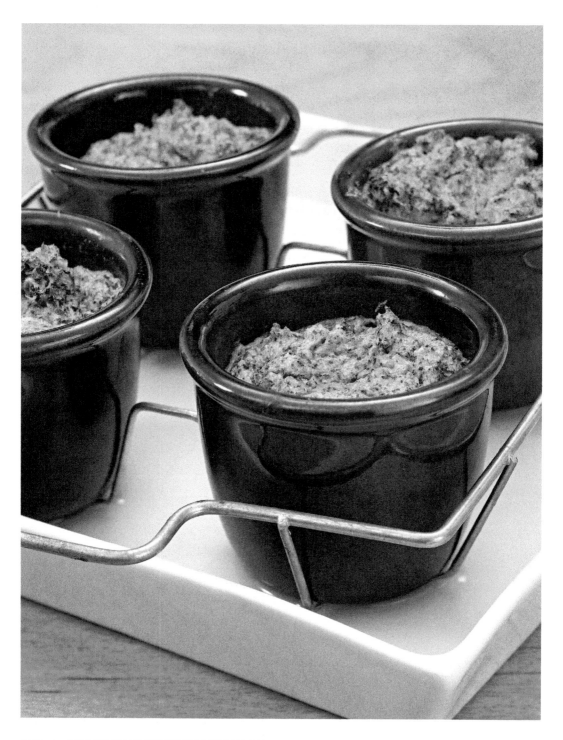

Balanced Broccoli Timbales

Broccoli is a rich source of fiber, beta-carotene, and vitamin C, and it is also a good source of calcium, making it helpful in fighting arthritis and osteoporosis. With the addition of crème fraiche and eggs, this dish provides a good balance of healthy fat and protein and is great for any occasion.

INGREDIENTS
12 ounces (340 g) broccoli florets, steamed
3 tablespoons (45 ml) crème fraiche or whipping cream
1 egg, plus 1 egg yolk
1 tablespoon (6 g) chopped scallions
Salt and freshly ground black pepper to taste
Pinch of grated nutmeg
Fresh chopped chives for garnish
Fresh chopped parsley for garnish
Hollandaise sauce (optional) (page 105)
1 teaspoon butter

Yield: 4 servings

Health Facilitators	Nutrient Density Rating
Protein	Moderate
Fat	Moderate
Carbohydrate	High
Enzymes	Moderate
Antioxidants	Very High
Fiber	Very High

Preheat oven to 375°F (190°C, or gas mark 5). Lightly butter four 4.5-ounce (135 ml) ramekins, and line bases with lightly buttered greaseproof paper.

Process the cooked broccoli in a food processor with cream, egg, and egg yolk until smooth. Add scallions, and season with salt, pepper, and nutmeg. Pulse to mix.

Spoon the purée into ramekins, place in a bain marie (a dish with water in it), and bake for 25 minutes or until just set. Invert ramekins onto warmed plates and peel off paper. Garnish abundantly with fresh parsley and chives. Serve with hollandaise sauce, if desired.

Did You Know?
Although raw broccoli is bursting with nutrients, cooked broccoli is actually better for you, because lightly steaming or stir-frying it releases its abundant phytochemicals and antioxidants.

Tofu and Peanut-Butter Stuffed Celery

Tofu has been called the perfect food. It is high in protein, calcium, and vitamin E and low in cholesterol. Sesame seeds help to protect the body from free radicals and are a key source of magnesium and calcium. This flavorful combination of sesame, peanuts, and lime, with a dash of spice from cayenne pepper, brings zest and a heavy dose of antioxidants to high-fiber celery.

INGREDIENTS

1 tablespoon (8 g) raw sesame seeds
½ pound (225 g) firm tofu, drained, pressed, and crumbled
3 tablespoons (48 g) peanut butter, creamy or crunchy (no sugar added)
1 tablespoon (15 g) sesame tahini
2 teaspoons low-sodium tamari soy sauce
1 tablespoon (15 ml) fresh lime juice
Dash cayenne pepper
6 celery stalks, cut into 2-inch (5-cm) pieces

Yield: 6 servings

Put sesame seeds in an ungreased skillet over medium-high heat. Stir seeds or shake pan almost constantly until seeds are evenly browned and toasted and begin to pop. Remove from pan immediately and set aside.

In a food processor, combine tofu, peanut butter, sesame tahini, soy sauce, lime juice, and cayenne pepper until creamy. Spoon into celery stalks and top with toasted sesame seeds.

Did You Know?

Celery has strong diuretic (water removing) powers, making it useful in the treatment of health problems such as arthritis and rheumatism. Sufferers may consume the vegetable raw, cooked, or juiced, which is the most effective form of all.

Health Facilitators	Nutrient Density Rating
Protein	High
Fat	Very High
Carbohydrate	High
Enzymes	High
Antioxidants	High
Fiber	High

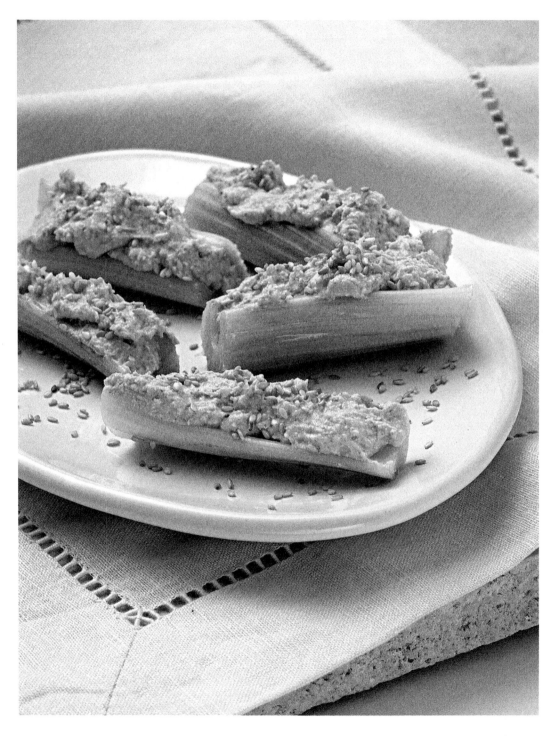

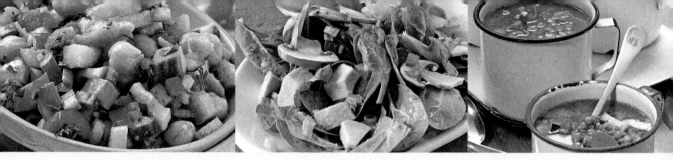

CHAPTER 9

FRESH AND LIVELY

Daily Fare Salad (RAW)

It's hard to beat the combination of flavors that come from the broad range of healthy ingredients in this main course salad. It is loaded with enzymes and a huge variety of anti-oxidants, minerals, and vitamins. This salad achieves its balance of healthy fats and protein from nuts and sunflower seeds, and it gets a spicy kick from radishes and red onions. Aim to have a salad like this every day—just tailor the ingredients to what's in season.

Ingredients
4 cups (220 g) mixed salad greens

Additions (choose at least 6):
½ cup (70 g) diced cucumbers
½ cup (60 g) sliced radishes
1 cup (90 g) shredded red cabbage
1 cup (116 g) shredded radicchio
½ cup (60 g) diced celery
1 cup (70 g) sliced brown
   or white mushrooms
½ cup (60 g) grated carrots
1 cup (150 g) thinly sliced red
   or green bell pepper
½ cup (45 g) thinly sliced fennel
½ (50 g) cup diced scallions
½ cup (80 g) thinly sliced red onion
¼ cup (35 g) raw sunflower seeds
¼ cup (30 g) chopped raw walnuts

Yield: 4 servings

In a large bowl, toss all ingredients and serve with your choice of dressing. (See Salad Dressings, page 160–168.)

Did You Know?
When it comes to health benefits and therapeutic value, cabbage is a superfood. It can kill certain viruses and bacteria, boost your immune and digestive systems, and help maintain the integrity of nerve endings.

Health Facilitators	Nutrient Density Rating
Protein	High
Fat	Moderate
Carbohydrate	High
Enzymes	High
Antioxidants	High
Fiber	High

Beta-Carrot Salad (RAW)

Enjoy the sunny flavors of carrots, herbs, and walnuts in this perfectly balanced, high-fiber dish. The beta-carotene in carrots is an antioxidant that converts to vitamin A, which helps strengthen your eyesight. Walnuts provide essential fatty acids that feed the brain and increase focus and concentration. You can't go wrong eating this delicious salad everyday

INGREDIENTS
For dressing
4 tablespoons (60 ml) fresh lime juice
1 teaspoon ground cumin
8 tablespoons (120 ml) pure-pressed
  extra-virgin olive oil
Freshly ground black pepper to taste

For salad
1 pound (454 g) shredded carrots
1 fennel bulb (stalk and core removed),
  cut lengthwise into thin strips
½ cup (60 g) chopped raw walnuts
½ cup (30 g) chopped fresh parsley

Yield: 4 servings

In a small bowl, using a fork, whisk together lime juice, cumin, and black pepper. Slowly drizzle in olive oil, whisking until smooth. Taste and adjust seasonings if neccessary.

In a separate bowl, combine carrots, fennel, walnuts, and parsley. Toss with dressing and marinate in refrigerator for one hour before serving.

Health Facilitators	Nutrient Density Rating
Protein	Moderate
Fat	High
Carbohydrate	Very High
Enzymes	High
Antioxidants	High
Fiber	High

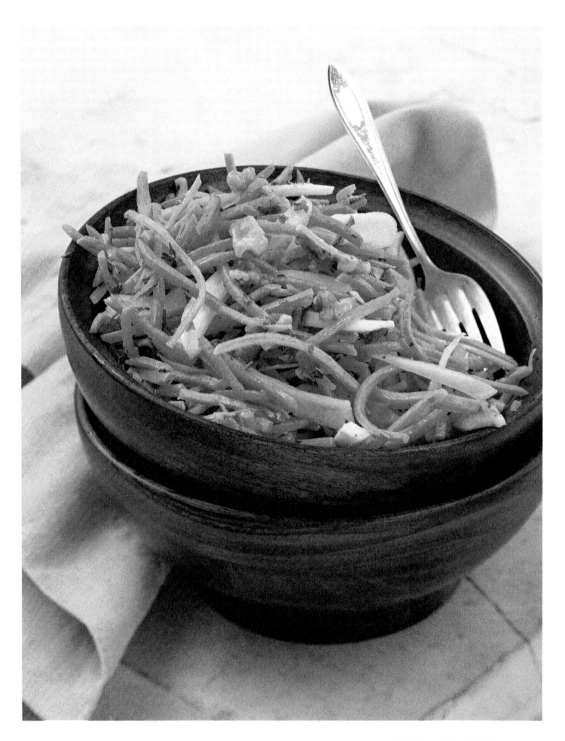

Lycopene Tomatoes with Mozzarella (RAW)

Enjoy the classic pairing of fresh tomatoes with mozzarella cheese and basil. Tomatoes contain a powerful antioxidant called lycopene that helps lower the risk of all cancers and reduces the risk of heart disease. They are also loaded with potassium, niacin, vitamin K, vitamin B6, and folate. Mozzarella cheese is a dense source of nutrients, including calcium and protein.

INGREDIENTS

For salad
4 large, very ripe tomatoes, thinly sliced
½ pound (225 g) fresh buffalo
   mozzarella cheese, thinly sliced
½ cup (20 g) fresh basil leaves,
   or 2 teaspoons dried basil

For vinaigrette
2 tablespoons (28 ml) red wine vinegar
3 tablespoons (45 ml) pure-pressed
   extra-virgin olive oil
Freshly ground black pepper to taste

Yield: 4 servings

Alternate slices of tomato, mozzarella, and fresh basil leaves on four plates. (If using dried basil, sprinkle on top.) In a small bowl, using a fork, whisk vinaigrette ingredients together until well blended. Spoon vinaigrette over salad. Refrigerate for one hour before serving.

Did You Know?
Tomatoes contain loads of vitamin C, which helps the body produce collagen—an important protein for skin, tendons, ligaments, and blood vessels.

Health Facilitators	Nutrient Density Rating
Protein	High
Fat	High
Carbohydrate	Very High
Enzymes	Very High
Antioxidants	Very High
Fiber	Very High

Bone-Building Cottage Cheese and Chopped Vegetable Salad (RAW)

Nutrient-dense cottage cheese combines well with fruits and vegetables, to pack an antioxidant punch. This dish contains vitamins A, C, E, and B6, folic acid, zinc, selenium, potassium, calcium, and magnesium—just a few nutrients that will boost your immune system and keep you strong. Don't spare the flax oil, to help fight inflammation and balance your hormones.

INGREDIENTS
4 cups (220 g) mixed salad greens
2 carrots, finely diced
3 scallions, finely chopped
1 small red bell pepper, finely chopped
3 celery stalks, finely chopped
2 tablespoons (8 g) fresh parsley, minced
1 tablespoon (3 g) fresh chives, minced
2 cups (450 g) whole-milk cottage cheese
2 tablespoons (28 ml) flaxseed oil
Freshly ground black pepper to taste
Dash cayenne pepper

Yield: 4 servings

Arrange mixed salad greens on 4 individual plates. In a medium bowl, using a fork, mix remaining ingredients with cottage cheese. Mound cottage cheese salad on mixed greens. Serve immediately.

Did You Know?
In the 1950s, Dr. Johanna Budwig, a German biochemist and expert on fats and oils, put forth the theory that a scientific oil-protein diet of flaxseed oil and organic cottage cheese was beneficial in preventing and even curing cancer. This combination was later re-examined by oncologist and cardiologist Dr. Dan C. Roehm who, in 1990, claimed, "This diet is far and away the most successful anti-cancer diet in the world."

Health Facilitators	Nutrient Density Rating
Protein	High
Fat	High
Carbohydrate	Very High
Enzymes	Very High
Antioxidants	Very High
Fiber	Very High

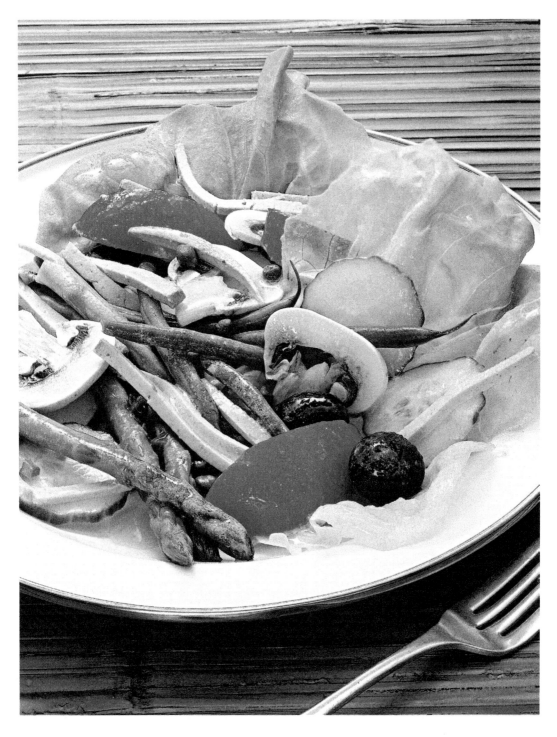

Salad Niçoise (RAW)

Make a perfectly balanced nutrient-dense meal out of this salad. It gets carbohydrates from potatoes, green beans, and asparagus, which are high in vitamin C, potassium, calcium, magnesium, zinc, and folic acid. You get protein from the tofu, and you can get even more by adding canned salmon or tuna. Plenty of fresh greens and the garden's finest vegetables combine to create a giant serving of enzymes, fiber, and antioxidants.

INGREDIENTS

1 head Bibb or green leaf lettuce, washed and dried
2 red potatoes, steamed and sliced into ¼-inch (6-mm) rounds
24 fresh green beans, steamed 3 to 4 minutes, and rinsed in ice water
16 fresh asparagus spears, steamed 3 to 4 minutes, and rinsed in ice water
2 small ripe tomatoes, quartered
4 mushrooms, washed, dried, and sliced paper thin
½ cucumber, sliced
4 to 6 ounces (120 to 175 g) tofu, julienned
12 Niçoise or Greek olives, pitted
1 tablespoon (9 g) capers
Dijon Dressing (page 160)

Yield: 4 servings

Prepare each salad individually, laying down a flat bed of lettuce and attractively grouping each vegetable on top. Sprinkle capers on potatoes. Gently pour Dijon dressing over each salad just prior to serving. Serve at room temperature.

Health Facilitators	Nutrient Density Rating
Protein	Very High
Fat	Moderate
Carbohydrate	Very High
Enzymes	Very High
Antioxidants	Very High
Fiber	Very High

Energy Salad with Peanut Coconut Sauce

You will reap the numerous benefits of coconut oil from this dish. Coconut provides an immediate source of energy and supports a healthy immune system and metabolism. It keeps your skin and hair healthy and youthful-looking and promotes weight loss. You'll love the tasty flavors and the energy boost this delicious salad provides.

INGREDIENTS

For sauce
Olive-oil cooking spray,
   or ½ teaspoon toasted sesame oil
2 garlic cloves, peeled and minced
¼ teaspoon fresh chili peppers,
   minced, or chili paste
1 tablespoon (15 ml) lime or lemon juice
Himalayan crystal salt to taste
¾ cup (175 ml) coconut milk

For salad
1 large bunch fresh baby spinach,
   washed thoroughly, blotted or spun dry,
   and torn into pieces
½ cup (75 g) dry-roasted peanuts,
   finely ground

Yield: 4 servings

Heat a skillet to medium and season with oil. Sauté garlic gently for 2 to 3 minutes and remove skillet from heat. Add remaining sauce ingredients and stir to mix.

Toss together spinach and sauce. Garnish with dry-roasted peanuts. Serve immediately.

Did You Know?
Spinach is not only rich in iron to keep you strong, it also has vitamins A, C, and E, and some B vitamins, and it is a good source of fiber and protein.

Health Facilitators	Nutrient Density Rating
Protein	High
Fat	High
Carbohydrate	Very High
Enzymes	Very High
Antioxidants	Very High
Fiber	Very High

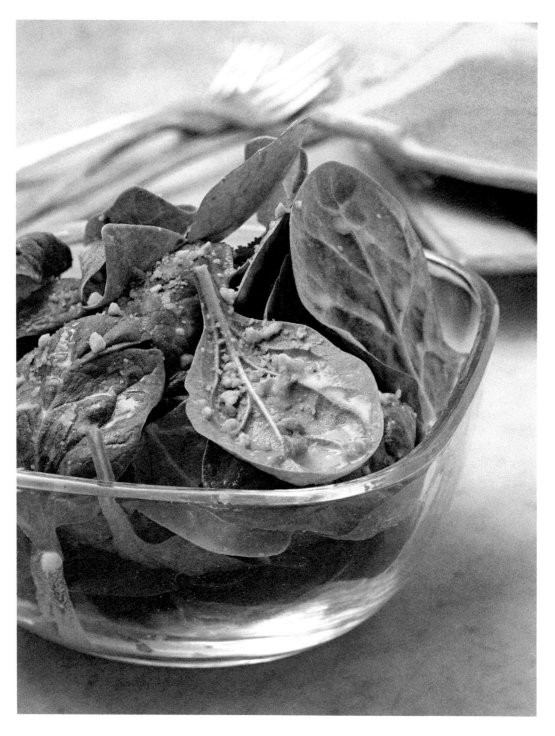

Calming Sweet Potato, Asparagus, Red Pepper, and Feta Cheese Salad

Sweet potatoes are the richest low-fat source of vitamin E. They are also loaded with beta-carotene and potassium. These nutrients protect against heart attack and stroke, maintain nerve function and blood pressure, and protect against inflammatory conditions.

INGREDIENTS

2 pounds (908 g) sweet potatoes
2 tablespoons (28 ml) pure-pressed
  extra-virgin olive oil
2 garlic cloves, peeled and minced
Freshly ground black pepper to taste
2 red bell peppers, roasted, or ¾ cup
  (135 g) store-bought roasted red bell
  peppers
1 pound (454 g) asparagus, sliced
  diagonally into 1-inch (2.5-cm) pieces
1 cup (120 g) diced celery stalks
Dash cayenne pepper
½ cup (20 g) slivered fresh basil
  or 2 teaspoons dried basil
½ cup (75 g) crumbled feta cheese
4 cups (220 g) mixed salad greens
Roasted Salad Dressing (page 160)

Yield: 6 servings

Preheat oven to 400°F (200°C, or gas mark 6). Peel potatoes and cut into 1-inch (2.5-cm) cubes. Toss with olive oil, garlic, and black pepper. Spread potatoes evenly over a lightly greased baking sheet. Roast until browned and tender, about 20 to 30 minutes, turning occasionally. Set aside.

If using fresh red bell peppers, roast peppers directly over a gas flame or under a preheated broiler on a broiler rack. Using tongs, turn peppers frequently until blistered and blackened on all sides. Place peppers in a bowl with a plate on top. Let steam for 15 minutes to loosen skins. Peel off charred skin and discard. Slice peppers in half and remove seeds. Cut roasted flesh into slivers. Set aside.

Cook asparagus until just barely tender by immersing into boiling water for 3 to 6 minutes. Drain, rinse under cold water, and drain again. Gently toss roasted potatoes with bell peppers, asparagus, celery, and cayenne pepper. Add fresh basil and crumbled feta cheese. Toss with Roasted Salad Dressing. Serve on a bed of salad greens.

Health Facilitators	Nutrient Density Rating
Protein	High
Fat	Moderate
Carbohydrate	Very High
Enzymes	Very High
Antioxidants	Very High
Fiber	Very High

Slimming Asparagus Salad with Dijon Vinaigrette (RAW)

With its diuretic properties from a high potassium and low sodium content, together with active amino acids, asparagus is great for relieving water retention and slimming down. It is rich in antioxidants, such as beta-carotene and vitamin C, as well as potassium and phosphorus for healthy heart and nervous system function. You'll enjoy it with the tasty addition of a tangy lime and mustard dressing.

INGREDIENTS

For vinaigrette

½ tablespoon (7.5 ml) lime juice
  or red wine vinegar
1 tablespoon (15 ml) pure-pressed
  extra-virgin olive oil
1 tablespoon (15 ml) purified water
1 clove garlic, peeled and crushed
1 teaspoon shallots, minced
1 teaspoon Dijon-style prepared mustard
$1/8$ teaspoon dry mustard
¼ teaspoon Himalayan crystal salt
Freshly ground black pepper

For salad

1 large bunch fresh asparagus
  (about 2½ pounds [1.2 kg])
½ head green leaf lettuce,
  washed and dried

Yield: 4 servings

Prepare dressing by blending vinaigrette ingredients together, then set aside. Wash and trim bottom ends of asparagus. Remove skins with a potato peeler, beginning halfway down stalk to ends. Marinate asparagus in dressing for 1 to 2 hours in an airtight container in the refrigerator. Serve asparagus chilled, on a bed of green leaf lettuce.

Health Facilitators	Nutrient Density Rating
Protein	High
Fat	Moderate
Carbohydrate	Very High
Enzymes	Very High
Antioxidants	Very High
Fiber	Very High

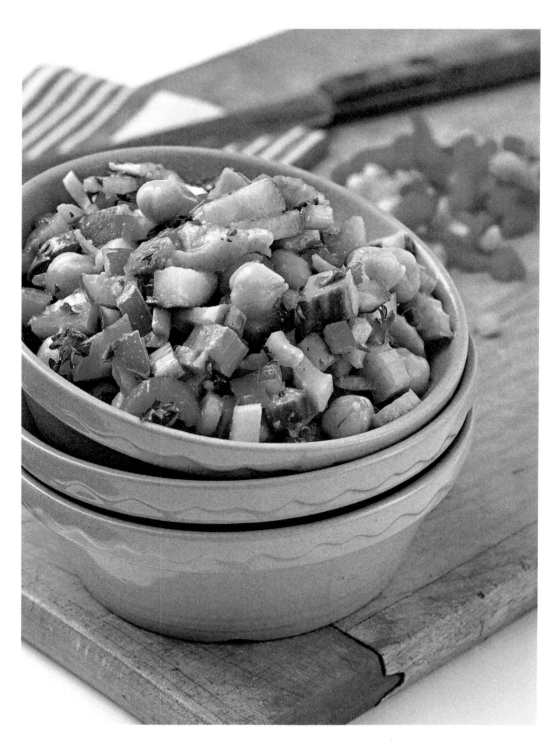

Pumping Jumping Bean Salad (RAW)

Garbanzo beans (also known as chickpeas) have a deliciously nutty taste and buttery texture. They will pump you full of protein for building strong muscles. Garbanzos can be enjoyed year-round and are high in fiber to keep blood sugar levels stable. With carrots, parsley, celery, and other goodies, this dish is loaded with vitamins, minerals, fiber, and antioxidants, to keep you fit and jumping.

INGREDIENTS

13¾-ounce (425-ml) can of
  garbanzo beans, drained and rinsed
½ cup (80 g) chopped red onion
1 cup (120 g) diced celery stalks
1 cup (130 g) diced carrot
½ cup (30 g) minced fresh parsley
1 cup (135 g) seeded and diced cucumber
1 cup (150 g) diced red bell pepper
Garbanzo Vinaigrette (page 161)

Yield: 4 servings

Combine all ingredients in a large bowl and toss with Garbanzo Vinaigrette. Cover, and chill for 1 hour before serving.

Health Facilitators	Nutrient Density Rating
Protein	Very High
Fat	Moderate
Carbohydrate	Very High
Enzymes	Very High
Antioxidants	Very High
Fiber	Very High

Avocado Advantage with Spinach and Mushrooms (RAW)

Creamy, rich avocado is considered the world's healthiest fruit because of its long list of nutrients: vitamin K, most of the B vitamins, some E and C, potassium, magnesium, iron, and dietary fiber. Spinach is loaded with iron and antioxidants, such as vitamin A and vitamin C.

INGREDIENTS
1 pound (454 g) fresh spinach leaves, washed, dried and torn into bite-size pieces
2 ripe avocados, peeled, diced, and sprinkled with juice from half a lemon
8 ounces (225 g) thinly sliced brown or white mushrooms
¼ cup (25 g) diced scallions
Garlic Dijon Vinaigrette (page 162)

Yield: 4 servings

In a large serving bowl, toss together all ingredients. Add Garlic Dijon Vinaigrette and serve immediately.

Did You Know?
Avocados help guard against circulatory diseases, such as heart disease, stroke, and high blood pressure.

Health Facilitators	Nutrient Density Rating
Protein	Moderate
Fat	High
Carbohydrate	High
Enzymes	Very High
Antioxidants	Very High
Fiber	Very High

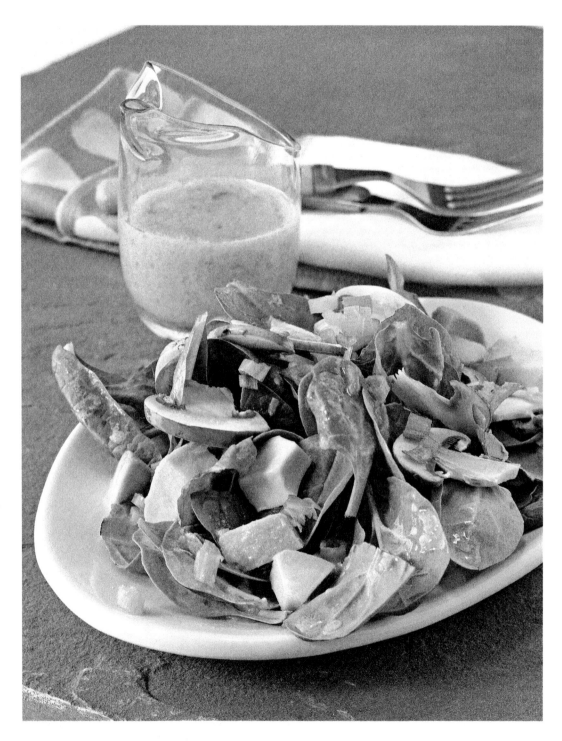

Dijon Dressing (RAW)

This dressing pairs perfectly with the Salad Niçoise on page 151.

INGREDIENTS

Juice of 1 lime
1 tablespoon (15 ml) pure-pressed
    extra-virgin olive oil
1 tablespoon (15 ml) flaxseed oil
3 tablespoons (45 ml) water
1 clove garlic, peeled and minced
1 to 2 teaspoons shallots, minced
1 teaspoon Dijon-style prepared mustard
¼ teaspoon dry mustard
Himalayan crystal salt and freshly ground
    pepper to taste

Yield: ½ cup (120 ml)

Whisk all ingredients together in a bowl.

Health Facilitators	Nutrient Density Rating
Protein	Low
Fat	Moderate
Carbohydrate	Moderate
Enzymes	High
Antioxidants	High
Fiber	Low

Roasted Salad Dressing (RAW)

This dressing is perfect for the veggie salad on page 145.

INGREDIENTS

2 tablespoons (28 ml) balsamic vinegar
2 teaspoons Dijon mustard
1 garlic clove, peeled and minced
4 tablespoons (60 ml) pure-pressed
    extra-virgin olive oil
2 tablespoons (30 ml) flaxseed oil
Freshly ground black pepper to taste

Yield: ½ cup (120 ml)

Whisk all ingredients together in a bowl.

Health Facilitators	Nutrient Density Rating
Protein	Low
Fat	Moderate
Carbohydrate	Moderate
Enzymes	High
Antioxidants	High
Fiber	Low

Garbanzo Vinaigrette (RAW)

This dressing is perfect for the Pumping Jumping Bean Salad on page 157. Don't spare the garlic and feel free to add a pinch of cayenne for some added zing.

INGREDIENTS
1 garlic clove, peeled and minced
4 tablespoons (60 ml) pure-pressed
extra-virgin olive oil
2 to 4 tablespoons (30 to 60 ml)
flaxseed oil
2 tablespoons (28 ml) fresh lemon juice
2 tablespoons (28 ml) balsamic vinegar
1 tablespoon (15 g) Dijon mustard
Freshly ground black pepper to taste

Yield: 1 cup (235 ml)

In a blender or food processor, combine all ingredients and blend until smooth, or place ingredients in a jar with a tight-fitting lid and shake vigorously until well blended. Taste, and adjust seasonings.

Health Facilitators	Nutrient Density Rating
Protein	Low
Fat	Moderate
Carbohydrate	Moderate
Enzymes	High
Antioxidants	High
Fiber	Low

Anti-Inflammatory Garlic Dijon Vinaigrette (RAW)

This mustard and garlic dressing gives a spicy, aromatic taste and fragrance to your salads and meals. Mustard seeds are a very good source of selenium, a nutrient that has been shown to reduce some symptoms associated with rheumatoid arthritis. They are also a good source of omega-3 essential fatty acids, as well as iron, calcium, zinc, magnesium, niacin, and protein. Bon appetit!

INGREDIENTS

3 tablespoons (45 ml) balsamic vinegar
¾ cup (175 ml) pure-pressed
  extra-virgin olive oil
2 garlic cloves, peeled and minced
1 tablespoon (11 g) mustard seeds, or
  1 tablespoon (15 g) prepared Dijon
  mustard
1 tablespoon (2.5 g) slivered fresh basil,
  or 1 teaspoon dried basil
Freshly ground black pepper to taste

Yield: 1 cup (235 ml)

In a blender or food processor, combine all ingredients and blend until smooth, or place ingredients in a jar with a tight-fitting lid and shake vigorously until well blended. Taste, and adjust seasonings.

Health Facilitators	Nutrient Density Rating
Protein	Low
Fat	Moderate
Carbohydrate	Low
Enzymes	High
Antioxidants	High
Fiber	High

Fighting-Fit Flaxseed Oil and Ginger Dressing (RAW)

Flaxseed oil is considered one of the richest sources of omega-3s, which makes it an excellent defense against degenerative disease and illness, including cardiovascular, cancer, kidney, auto-immune, bone, and joint problems. This dressing is nothing but good news.

INGREDIENTS
1 lemon, peeled, cut in half, and seeds removed
½ cup (120 ml) flaxseed oil
¼ cup (60 ml) pure-pressed extra-virgin olive oil
½ to 1 teaspoon fresh minced ginger
1 teaspoon Himalayan crystal salt
Freshly ground black pepper to taste
1 clove garlic (optional)

Yield: 1 cup (235 ml)

In a blender or food processor, combine all ingredients and blend until smooth and creamy. Taste, and adjust seasonings.

Did You Know?
Ginger has been used for more than 2,000 years in Chinese medicine to treat a number of health problems, including arthritis, rheumatism, sore throats, abdominal bloating, and indigestion.

Health Facilitators	Nutrient Density Rating
Protein	Low
Fat	Moderate
Carbohydrate	Low
Enzymes	High
Antioxidants	High
Fiber	Low

Soothing Dill and Lemon Dressing (RAW)

The dill plant, a relative of parsley, is valued for its delicate flavor and calming properties. It's helpful for overcoming insomnia and for soothing an upset stomach. Tahini makes this dressing an especially good source of calcium, protein, and B vitamins. Add lemons, which are loaded with antioxidants and build immune strength, and this dressing complements any fish dish, or you can drizzle it over steamed vegetables or fresh greens.

INGREDIENTS
½ cup (120 ml) flax oil
¼ cup (60 ml) pure-pressed
   extra-virgin olive oil
½ cup (120 ml) lemon juice
1 tablespoon (15 g) sesame tahini
2 teaspoons fresh dill
½ teaspoon Himalayan crystal salt
Freshly ground black pepper, to taste
1 clove garlic (optional)

Yield: 1 cup (235 ml)

In a blender or food processor, combine all ingredients and blend until smooth and creamy. Taste, and adjust seasonings.

Health Facilitators	Nutrient Density Rating
Protein	Moderate
Fat	High
Carbohydrate	High
Enzymes	High
Antioxidants	Very High
Fiber	Low

Tahini Lemon Dressing (RAW)

Sesame seeds contain two unique substances: *sesamin* and *sesamolin*. Both substances belong to a group of beneficial fibers called lignans, and they have been shown to have a cholesterol-lowering effect in humans and to prevent high blood pressure and increase vitamin E supplies in animals. Sesamin has also been found to protect the liver from oxidative damage.

INGREDIENTS

¾ cup (175 ml) purified or spring water
2 tablespoons (30 g) raw tahini
1 tablespoon (15 ml) lemon juice
1 teaspoon Himalayan crystal salt
1 teaspoon fresh chives
1 clove garlic, peeled and crushed
  (optional)
1 teaspoon fresh dill (optional)

Yield: 1 cup (235 ml)

In a blender or food processor, combine all ingredients and blend until smooth and creamy. Taste, and adjust seasonings.

Did You Know?
Sesame seeds are not only a good source of manganese and copper, they also have plenty of calcium, magnesium, iron, phosphorous, vitamin B1, zinc, and dietary fiber.

Health Facilitators	Nutrient Density Rating
Protein	High
Fat	High
Carbohydrate	Moderate
Enzymes	High
Antioxidants	High
Fiber	Low

Caesar Dressing with Heart (RAW)

Avocados deliver almost twenty vitamins, minerals, and beneficial phytonutrients, making them nutrient dense, heart healthy, and a satisfying addition to any healthy diet. This dressing starts with avocados and adds lemon juice for extra vitamin C, flaxseed oil for essential fatty acids, and cayenne pepper for a fiery zip. This one is especially good for your circulation and your heart.

INGREDIENTS

3 avocados, peeled and pit removed
$^1/_3$ cup (80 ml) lemon juice
1 tablespoon (6 g) freshly ground
   black pepper
1 teaspoon Himalayan crystal salt
3 tablespoons (45 ml) pure-pressed
   extra-virgin olive oil
2 tablespoons (28 ml) flaxseed oil
¼ cup (60 ml) filtered water
1 teaspoon cayenne pepper

Yield: 2 cups (475 ml)

Combine all ingredients together in a high-powered blender and blend until creamy.

Did You Know?

Cayenne pepper is considered to be the number one herb for increasing your blood flow and aiding circulation. Cayenne also soothes the digestive tract and stimulates the flow of stomach secretions and saliva. These secretions contain substances which help digest food.

Health Facilitators	Nutrient Density Rating
Protein	Low
Fat	Very High
Carbohydrate	High
Enzymes	High
Antioxidants	Very High
Fiber	Low

Coconut Curry Dressing (RAW)

Coconuts boost immune-system function, fight aging, and promote good cholesterol. Avocados and coconuts are both excellent sources of essential fatty acids and nutrient-dense sources of many important vitamins, minerals, and antioxidants. This dressing is enhanced by an infusion of flavor from the curry powder and other herbs.

INGREDIENTS

2 cups (475 ml) coconut water
  (from fresh coconut)
1 cup (about 70 g) coconut pulp
  (from fresh coconut)
½ avocado, peeled and pit removed
1 tablespoon (15 ml) lemon juice
1 tablespoon (7 g) curry powder
1 teaspoon ground cumin
1 teaspoon ground coriander
1 teaspoon Himalayan crystal salt

Yield: 2½ cups (570 ml)

In a blender or food processor, combine all ingredients and blend until smooth and creamy. Taste, and adjust seasonings.

Did You Know?

Coconut water is identical to human blood plasma, which makes up 55 percent of human blood, making it the perfect universal donor. During the Pacific War (1941–1945), coconut water was actually used to give emergency plasma transfusions to wounded soldiers, as it is also a sterile solution, does not produce heat, does not destroy red blood cells, and is readily accepted by the body.

Health Facilitators	Nutrient Density Rating
Protein	Moderate
Fat	Very High
Carbohydrate	Low
Enzymes	High
Antioxidants	Very High
Fiber	Moderate

Cleansing Cilantro Lime Dressing

This dressing is loaded with immune-boosting phytonutrients, vitamins, and minerals. Cilantro, the leaves of the coriander plant, helps your body to remove—or chelate—toxic metals, such as mercury, lead, and aluminum, from the nervous system and body tissue. Take advantage of the cleansing powers of this "poor man's chelation therapy" by adding a small amount of cilantro to your daily diet for two or three weeks.

INGREDIENTS
8 tablespoons (112 g) unsalted butter
½ cup (80 g) chopped red onion
2 minced garlic cloves
3 tablespoons (45 ml) fresh lime juice
2 teaspoons grated lime zest
Dash hot pepper sauce
2 tablespoons (8 g) chopped fresh
  cilantro
Freshly ground black pepper to taste

Yield: 1 cup (235 ml)

Health Facilitators	Nutrient Density Rating
Protein	None
Fat	Moderate
Carbohydrate	High
Enzymes	High
Antioxidants	High
Fiber	Low

In a medium frying pan or skillet, melt butter over medium-high heat. When butter is hot and bubbling, add onion and garlic, and cook until softened, about 5 minutes. Add lime juice, zest, hot-pepper sauce, cilantro, and black pepper. Simmer 5 minutes over medium-low heat. Transfer to a blender or food processor and blend until smooth. Taste, and adjust seasonings. Serve immediately over steamed vegetables or rice dishes, or refrigerate and use cold in salads.

Did You Know?
Limes are an excellent source of vitamin C, one of the main antioxidants found in nature. They are packed with phytonutrients known as flavonoids—compounds that have antioxidant and anti-cancer properties—and are known for their antibiotic effect.

Soul-Warming Vegetable Stock

Adding sea vegetables to this stock enriches it with health-producing minerals from the ocean. The stock will have a little oil from the walnuts and olive oil; don't remove it, because it provides essential fatty acids.

INGREDIENTS

For stock

1 large onion, peeled and cut up
2 carrots, cut into chunks
2 celery stalks, cut into ½-inch pieces
1 medium leek, cleaned and sliced
1 turnip, cut into medium dice
10 mushrooms with stems, sliced
¼ cup (30 g) walnuts
1½ tablespoons (25 ml) pure-pressed
    extra-virgin olive oil
1 piece kombu seaweed
    (about 5 inches [12.5 cm])
¼ cup (55 g) dried white beans, soaked
    for 8 hours and drained
4 quarts (3.8 L) cold filtered water
2 garlic cloves, peeled
¼ cup (15 g) parsley stems (no leaves)
1 bay leaf
1 teaspoon sage, fresh or dried
1 teaspoon thyme, fresh or dried
½ teaspoon peppercorns

Piece of cheesecloth

Yield: 2 quarts (1.9 L)

Preheat oven to 450°F (230°C, or gas mark 8). Place the vegetables and walnuts in an 11×15-inch (28 × 38-cm) baking pan and coat with oil. Roast for about 20 minutes or until lightly browned. Turn vegetables every 5 to 6 minutes so they cook evenly.

Place the roasted vegetables, seaweed, white beans, and water into a 6- or 8-quart (5.7 or 7.6 L) stock pot. Add a little water to the baking pan to deglaze it and to loosen the brown bits and juices. Pour the contents of the pan into the stockpot. Place herbs for bouquet garnish on a 6 × 6-inch (15 × 15-cm) piece of cheesecloth and tie into a bundle; add to the pot.

Bring to a boil, then simmer for 1 hour with the cover slightly ajar. Make sure stock simmers very slowly—avoid a rolling boil. Remove the cover from the pot and simmer for 30 minutes more.

Discard the bouquet garni. Strain the stock.

Health Facilitators	Nutrient Density Rating
Protein	Low
Fat	Moderate
Carbohydrate	High
Enzymes	None
Antioxidants	High
Fiber	None

Super Vegetable Minestrone

Minestrone, made with an assortment of vegetables, including leeks, carrots, onions, celery, potatoes, tomatoes, and whole grain rice or beans, is a consistently good choice for any time of year or to have at any meal. It is loaded with vitamins, minerals, and antioxidants, and it's considered a "secret weapon" for improved health and weight loss. Cook up a large batch and have some every day to satisfy hunger and provide vital minerals and vitamins. This one is super good for you.

INGREDIENTS

1½ quarts (1.4 L) purified or spring water
1 strip kombu seaweed (optional)
½ to 1 cup (95 to 190 g) whole-grain
  brown rice, dried kidney beans, or
  lentils
1 tablespoon (2.4 g) fresh thyme,
  or ½ tablespoon (1.4 g) dried thyme
1 tablespoon (4 g) fresh marjoram,
  or ½ tablespoon (1 g) dried marjoram
2 leeks, cut into ½-inch (1.3-cm) pieces
1 small onion, peeled and chopped
2 large tomatoes, peeled and diced
1 potato, cut into cubes
2 celery stalks, chopped
3 carrots, cut into small pieces
1 cup (120 g) zucchini, chopped
1 cup (70 g) broccoli florets, chopped
1 cup (150 g) sweet peas
Salt to taste

Yield: 6 servings

Bring water, kombu, rice, and herbs (if using dried) to a boil, and simmer for 30 minutes. Add leeks, onion, tomatoes, potato, celery, carrots, and zucchini, and simmer 15 minutes longer. Add broccoli florets, sweet peas, and herbs (if using fresh), and simmer another 10 minutes. Remove kombu, salt to taste, and serve.

Health Facilitators	Nutrient Density Rating
Protein	High
Fat	Moderate
Carbohydrate	High
Enzymes	High
Antioxidants	High
Fiber	High

All-Season Vegetable and Split-Pea Soup

When fresh peas are not available, or when you want to enjoy a starchier, hardier-flavored legume, dried peas are the perfect alternative, because they are available at any time of the year. Dried peas, such as split-peas, are an excellent source of dietary fiber and a good source of protein, potassium, phosphorus, folate, and vitamin B1. This soup is a light, healthy meal for any time of day, to help you regenerate and energize your body.

INGREDIENTS

1 cup (225 g) split peas, rinsed
6 cups (1.4 L) vegetable stock or water
2 tablespoons (28 ml) pure-pressed
   extra-virgin olive oil
1 medium onion, finely chopped
2 garlic cloves, peeled and minced
2 celery stalks with leaves, diced
2 carrots, diced
1 teaspoon ground cumin
1 teaspoon dried oregano
2 bay leaves
2 tablespoons (8 g) minced fresh parsley
Freshly ground black pepper to taste
Dash red pepper flakes
1 to 2 tablespoons (15 to 28 ml)
   fresh lemon juice, or to taste

Yield: 6 servings

In a large heavy-bottomed soup pot, bring split peas and stock or water to a boil over high heat. Reduce heat to low, cover, and simmer for 30 minutes, skimming off any foam that collects on the surface.

In a large frying pan or skillet, heat oil over medium-high heat. When oil is hot, add onion, garlic, celery, carrots, cumin, oregano, bay leaves, parsley, black pepper, and red pepper flakes. Cook until vegetables have softened, about 8 minutes, stirring occasionally.

Add sautéed vegetables to soup pot and simmer, uncovered, for 1 hour, or until peas are soft, stirring occasionally. Remove bay leaves. In a blender or food processor, purée soup in batches until smooth. Add lemon juice to taste, and adjust seasonings.

Health Facilitators	Nutrient Density Rating
Protein	High
Fat	Low
Carbohydrate	High
Enzymes	Low
Antioxidants	Very High
Fiber	Very High

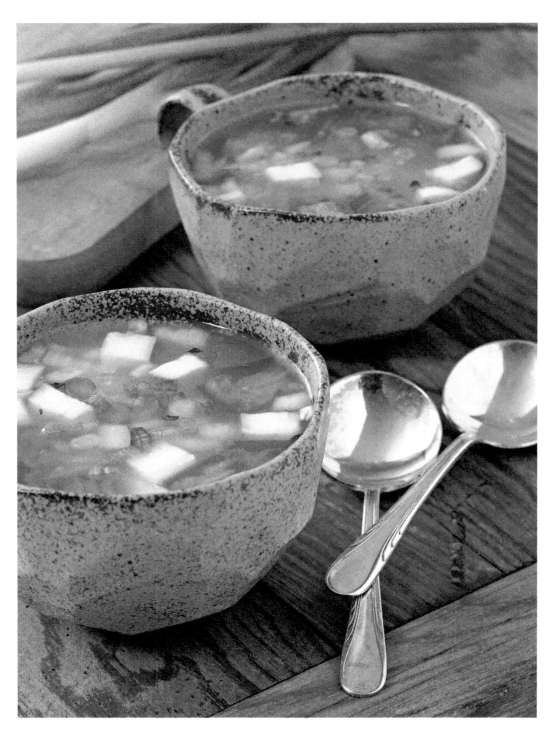

Virile Vegetable Soup

Enjoy the many health benefits of this deliciously thick and spicy vegetable soup. It is loaded with antioxidants and vitamin C for reducing stress and inflammation. To increase fiber and protein, add a bunch of chopped fresh spinach or a cup of whole grain brown rice or lentils, and you'll have a complete meal. This one is great for breakfast, lunch, or dinner. Enjoy!

INGREDIENTS

1 pound (454 g) small or medium potatoes
4 cups (946 ml) filtered water
¼ teaspoon cayenne pepper
½ teaspoon dried basil
½ teaspoon ground cumin
3 tablespoons (45 ml) sesame oil
Himalayan crystal salt to taste
½ cup (60 g) of each of the following:
    carrot, celery, green pepper, zucchini, broccoli, cauliflower, beets (for pink soup)
1 small onion, chopped
2 cloves garlic, peeled and chopped (optional)
½ cup (90 g) tomato, diced
½ cup (50 g) chopped scallions

Yield: 4 servings

Scrub potatoes and place in a medium-sized pot or sauce pan with 4 cups (946 ml) water. Boil for 15 to 20 minutes and allow to cool slightly. Put potatoes and their cooking water in a blender and mix with the cayenne pepper, basil, cumin, sesame oil, and salt to taste. Rinse vegetables and chop into bite-sized pieces. Place blended mixture and chopped vegetables into the pot or saucepan. Add onion, garlic, and tomato, and cook, covered, over low heat, for 10 to 15 minutes. Top with chopped scallions and serve.

Health Facilitators	Nutrient Density Rating
Protein	Low
Fat	Low
Carbohydrate	Very High
Enzymes	Low
Antioxidants	Very High
Fiber	Moderate

Healing Cream of Mushroom Soup

Mushrooms provide a wealth of protein, fiber, B vitamins, and vitamin C, as well as calcium and other minerals. And at least three mushroom varieties have demonstrated phenomenal healing power: maitake, shiitake, and reishi. These medicinal mushrooms have been shown to boost heart health, lower the risk of cancer, promote immune function, reduce inflammation, and support the body's detoxification mechanisms. So eat up!

INGREDIENTS

2 tablespoons (28 g) unsalted butter
1 cup (160 g) onion, minced
1 garlic clove, peeled and minced
1 pound (454 g) thinly sliced maitake, shiitake, or reishi mushrooms
1 tablespoon (8 g) flour
4 cups (946 ml) vegetable stock
1 tablespoon (4 g) fresh parsley, finely chopped
1 bay leaf
¼ teaspoon nutmeg, or ½ teaspoon dried thyme
Dash cayenne pepper
1 cup (235 ml) heavy cream
4 sprigs fresh parsley for garnish

Yield: 4 servings

In a large heavy-bottomed soup pot, melt butter over medium-high heat. When butter is hot and bubbling, add onion and garlic and sauté until softened, about 5 minutes. Add mushrooms and cook until they release their liquid and soften, about 5 minutes.

Sprinkle flour over onion and mushroom mixture, and cook over low heat, stirring, 3 to 4 minutes. Gradually add stock, parsley, bay leaf, nutmeg or thyme, and cayenne pepper. Bring to a boil, stirring constantly. Reduce heat and simmer gently for 20 minutes, stirring occasionally. Stir in cream. Simmer until heated through. Do not boil.

Taste, and adjust seasonings. Garnish each bowl with a sprig of fresh parsley.

Health Facilitators	Nutrient Density Rating
Protein	High
Fat	Low
Carbohydrate	High
Enzymes	Low
Antioxidants	High
Fiber	High

Creamy Tomato Soup (RAW)

The addition of avocado to lycopene-laden tomatoes packs this creamy soup with phytonutrients and antioxidants. To enhance the nutritional value of the lycopene, add half a teaspoon of olive oil. This soup is lovely sprinkled with fresh parsley and served with flax crackers.

INGREDIENTS

3 tomatoes

1 avocado

½ cup (68 g) macadamia nuts, soaked overnight in purified or spring water

½ cup (28 g) sun-dried tomatoes (dry-packed not oil-packed), soaked in 1½ cups (355 ml) water

½ teaspoon Himalayan crystal salt

½ teaspoon fresh chopped basil

½ teaspoon pure-pressed extra-virgin olive oil

2 to 3 tablespoons (8 to 12 g) fresh chopped parsley

Yield: 4 servings

In a blender, mix all ingredients until smooth. Refrigerate until cold. Serve with flax crackers and garnished with chopped parsley.

Did You Know?

Lycopene, found primarily in tomatoes, is a known cancer-fighting substance that comes from the carotenoids family, which includes beta-carotene and similar compounds found naturally in food. Research from the *Journal of the National Cancer Institute* found tremendous consistency among seventy-two different studies which showed that the more tomatoes and tomato products an individual consumes, the lower the rate of cancer, particularly cancers of the prostate, lung, and stomach.

Health Facilitators	Nutrient Density Rating
Protein	Low
Fat	Moderate
Carbohydrate	High
Enzymes	Very High
Antioxidants	Very High
Fiber	High

Balancing Curry and Lentil Soup

Lentils, like beans, are a good source of protein. They also provide calcium, phosphorus, vitamin B, and iron. They combine well with rice, beans, and vegetables such as carrots and zucchini, and of course, they make terrific lentil soup.

INGREDIENTS

3 tablespoons (45 g) unsalted butter
1 large onion, diced
2 garlic cloves, peeled and minced
1 green or red bell pepper, diced
2 celery stalks with leaves, diced
2 carrots, diced
2 zucchini, quartered lengthwise, and
   diced into ½-inch (1.3-cm) cubes
1 teaspoon ground cumin
1 teaspoon curry powder
2 cups (385 g) lentils, picked over and
   rinsed
8 cups (1.9 L) vegetable stock
1 bay leaf
1 tablespoon (6 g) fresh ginger,
   peeled and finely minced
1 cup (180 g) diced tomatoes
2 tablespoons (8 g) finely chopped
   fresh cilantro
Freshly ground black pepper to taste
1 tablespoon (15 ml) fresh lemon juice

Yield: 8 servings

In a large heavy-bottomed soup pot, melt butter over medium-high heat. When butter is hot and bubbling, add onion, garlic, and bell pepper and cook until softened, about 5 minutes. Add celery, carrots, zucchini, cumin, and curry powder and sauté for 5 minutes. Add lentils, stock, and bay leaf. Bring to a boil, reduce heat, and simmer over low heat, covered, for 30 to 45 minutes, or until lentils are tender. Add ginger, tomatoes, cilantro, and black pepper. Simmer another 15 minutes to blend flavors. Stir in lemon juice. Taste, and adjust seasonings.

Did You Know?

Because lentils contain a large amount of fiber, they are effective in lowering cholesterol and managing blood sugar disorders, as well as helping to prevent heart disease.

Health Facilitators	Nutrient Density Rating
Protein	High
Fat	Low
Carbohydrate	High
Enzymes	Low
Antioxidants	High
Fiber	Very High

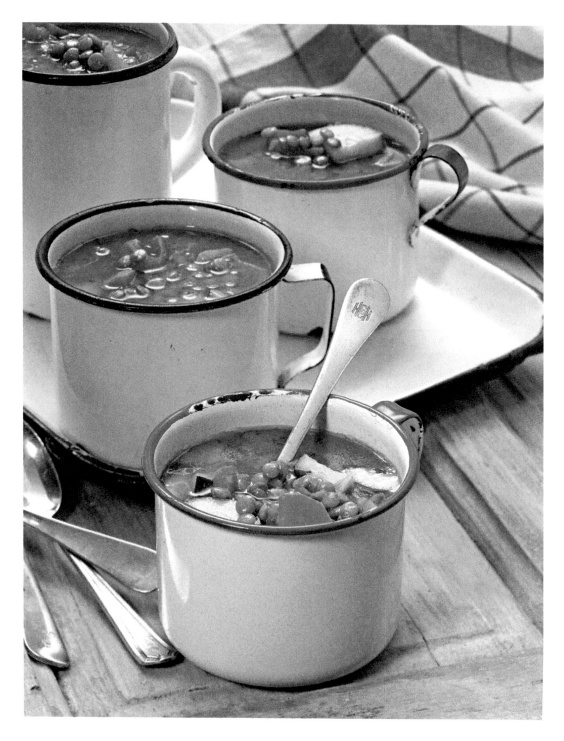

Stabilizing Black Bean Soup

Filled with fiber, iron, and magnesium, as well as loads of antioxidants, black beans are a wise choice for people with diabetes or hypoglycemia, because they stabilize blood sugar levels.

INGREDIENTS

2 cups (500 g) dried black beans
2 tablespoons (28 ml) pure-pressed extra-virgin olive oil
1 medium red onion, chopped
3 garlic cloves, peeled and minced
1 green or red bell pepper, diced
½ cup (60 g) chopped celery
½ cup (65 g) diced carrots
1 teaspoon ground cumin
1 teaspoon chili powder
1 teaspoon dried oregano
2 bay leaves
14½-ounce (440-ml) can of tomatoes, chopped and peeled, with juice
Freshly ground black pepper to taste
3 tablespoons (12 g) finely chopped cilantro
Dash hot pepper sauce (optional)
1 to 2 tablespoons (15 to 28 ml) fresh lime juice to taste
½ cup (120 ml) whole-milk sour cream

Yield: 6 servings

Soak beans overnight by covering them with at least 4 inches (10 cm) of water. Drain and rinse well. Place beans in a large heavy-bottomed soup pot and cover with about 10 cups (2.3 L) of fresh water. Bring to a boil. Reduce heat to medium and cook, uncovered, until tender, about 45 minutes to one hour, skimming off any foam that collects on the surface.

In a large frying pan or skillet, heat oil over medium-high heat. When oil is hot, add red onion, garlic, bell pepper, celery, carrots, cumin, and chili powder, and sauté until vegetables are softened, about 8 minutes. Add oregano, bay leaves, and tomatoes and their juice. Stir well.

Add the sautéed vegetable mixture to the cooked beans and mix well. Cook over low heat for 30 minutes, stirring occasionally, until beans are soft. Add more water, if necessary. Remove bay leaves. Season to taste with black pepper. Stir in chopped cilantro, hot pepper sauce, and lime juice. Taste, and adjust seasonings. Blend until smooth in a blender or food processor, if desired. Serve with a spoonful of sour cream.

Health Facilitators	Nutrient Density Rating
Protein	Very High
Fat	Low
Carbohydrate	Moderate
Enzymes	Low
Antioxidants	High
Fiber	Very High

Satisfying Butternut Bisque

Butternut squash and carrots make a great team—they're sweet, soul-satisfying vegetables that compete with each other for beta-carotene content and a comforting, earthy flavor. This wholesome soup is high in antioxidants and can inhibit cancer cell development.

INGREDIENTS

2 tablespoons (28 ml) pure-pressed
   extra-virgin olive oil
1 medium onion, chopped
1 medium butternut squash
5 cups (1.2 L) vegetable stock
   or filtered water
½ teaspoon Himalayan crystal salt
¼ teaspoon ground cumin
¼ teaspoon coriander powder
¼ teaspoon ginger powder
¼ teaspoon garlic powder
3 large carrots, chopped
1 cup (60 g) parsley, chopped
6 tablespoons (90 g) yogurt
½ cup (60 g) toasted almonds,
   chopped, for garnish

Yield: 6 servings

Place olive oil in a pan, add the chopped onion, and cook for 2 to 3 minutes. Wash butternut squash, cut in half, scoop out seeds, and cut into 1-inch (2.5 cm) cubes. (Include the squash peel; many vitamins are found just beneath the surface of the skin.) Place squash in soup pot with stock or water, salt, and spices. Add chopped carrots. Bring to a boil and simmer, covered, until you can pierce the pieces easily with a fork, about 15 to 20 minutes.

Purée the soup in a blender or food processor with parsley. Serve with one tablespoon (15 g) of yogurt in each cup and a sprinkle of chopped toasted almonds.

Health Facilitators	Nutrient Density Rating
Protein	Low
Fat	Low
Carbohydrate	Very High
Enzymes	None
Antioxidants	Very High
Fiber	Very High

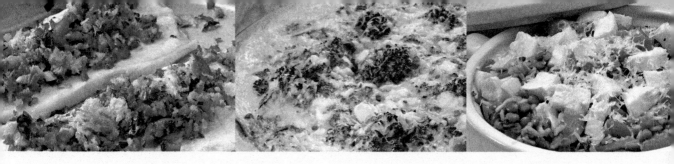

CHAPTER 10

SITTING DOWN TO DINNER

Baked Halibut with Corn Salsa

Halibut is truly a nutrient-dense food. An excellent source of high-quality protein, halibut is rich in significant amounts of a variety of important nutrients, including the minerals selenium, magnesium, phosphorus, and potassium; the vitamins B12, niacin, and B6; and perhaps most important, the beneficial omega-3 essential fatty acids. Corn is high in dietary fiber and vitamin C and is loaded with enzymes.

INGREDIENTS

1 cup (175 g) fresh or frozen corn kernels
½ cup (75 g) green pepper, seeded and diced
½ cup (75 g) red pepper, seeded and diced
½ medium onion, diced
$2/3$ cup (160 ml) plus 2 tablespoons (28 ml) freshly squeezed lemon juice
$2/3$ cup (160 ml) freshly squeezed lime juice
2 teaspoons chili pepper, seeded and diced
6 halibut fillets
1 tablespoon (15 ml) pure-pressed extra-virgin olive oil
Salsa
1 bunch fresh cilantro, finely chopped

Yield: 6 servings

In a small bowl, combine corn, green and red peppers, onion, $2/3$ cup (160 ml) lemon juice, lime juice, and chili pepper. Stir to mix well and chill in the refrigerator for at least 1 to 2 hours. Preheat oven to 350°F (180°C, or gas mark 4). Place halibut fillets in a large baking dish; sprinkle with olive oil and 2 tablespoons (28 ml) lemon juice. Bake for 15 to 20 minutes. Serve with salsa and fresh cilantro.

Health Facilitators	Nutrient Density Rating
Protein	Very High
Fat	Low
Carbohydrate	Low
Enzymes	Very High
Antioxidants	Very High
Fiber	High

Wild Mediterranean Dill Salmon

Wild salmon is a highly nutritious food. Of course, it is high in protein and the omega-3 essential fatty acids. But did you know that a four-ounce serving of wild salmon provides a full day's requirement of vitamin D? It is one of the few foods that can make that claim! That same piece of fish contains more than half our daily requirement of vitamin B12, niacin, and selenium and is an excellent source of vitamin B6 and magnesium.

INGREDIENTS
2 tablespoons (28 ml) soy sauce
2 tablespoons (28 ml) lemon or lime juice
6 wild salmon fillets
3 tablespoons (15 g) Parmesan cheese
6 lemon slices
6 tomato slices
6 sprigs fresh dill

Yield: 6 servings

Preheat oven to 375°F (190°C, or gas mark 5). Mix together soy sauce and lemon or lime juice; dip salmon fillets in mixture to coat both sides. Place the fillets in a large baking dish. Sprinkle with parmesan cheese, top with a lemon slice, a tomato slice, and a sprig of dill, and cover with lid or foil. Bake for about 20 minutes.

Did You Know?
Dill is a good source of calcium, dietary fiber, and the minerals manganese and iron. Dill's unique health benefits come from two types of phytonutrients: monoterpenes and flavonoids, both of which have antioxidant and anti-inflammatory properties.

Health Facilitators	Nutrient Density Rating
Protein	Very High
Fat	Low
Carbohydrate	Low
Enzymes	Low
Antioxidants	Very High
Fiber	Low

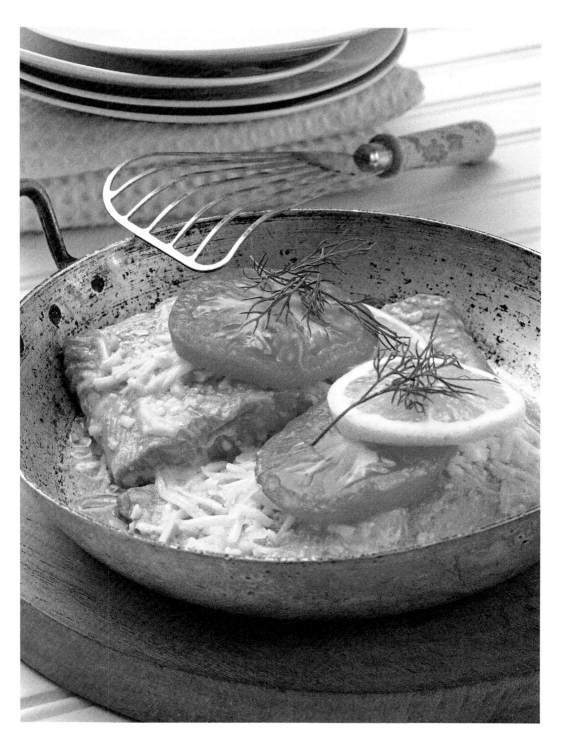

Baked Trout with Italian Herbs

In addition to its high-quality protein, fatty fish like trout is high in two kinds of omega-3 fatty acids: EPA and DHA, both of which are nourishing for your heart and your brain. This dish combines tasty herbs, including parsley, which is high in vitamins A and C, iron and calcium, with a whole lot of antioxidants from garlic and red peppers. It provides you with a full supply of everything you need to keep you healthy on every level.

INGREDIENTS

2 teaspoons pure-pressed extra-virgin olive oil
1 red pepper, seeded, and finely chopped
2 scallions, finely chopped
1 clove garlic, peeled, and minced
½ cup (30 g) Italian bread, crumbled into fine pieces
1 tablespoon (3 g) chives, chopped
1 tablespoon (4 g) fresh parsley, chopped
6 trout fillets
½ cup (115 g) mayonnaise or yogurt
6 lemon wedges
Salt and freshly ground black pepper to taste

Yield: 6 servings

Preheat oven to 375°F (190°C, or gas mark 5). In a large sauté pan, heat olive oil over medium heat and sauté red pepper for 5 minutes. Add scallions and garlic and continue to cook until soft. Remove pepper mixture from the heat and stir in the bread crumbs, chives, and parsley. Spread the top of the trout fillets with mayonnaise or yogurt. Sprinkle fillets with the crumb topping and bake for 15 to 20 minutes or until fish flakes easily with a fork. Season with salt and pepper and serve garnished with fresh lemon wedges.

Health Facilitators	Nutrient Density Rating
Protein	Very High
Fat	Low
Carbohydrate	Moderate
Enzymes	Very High
Antioxidants	Very High
Fiber	Moderate

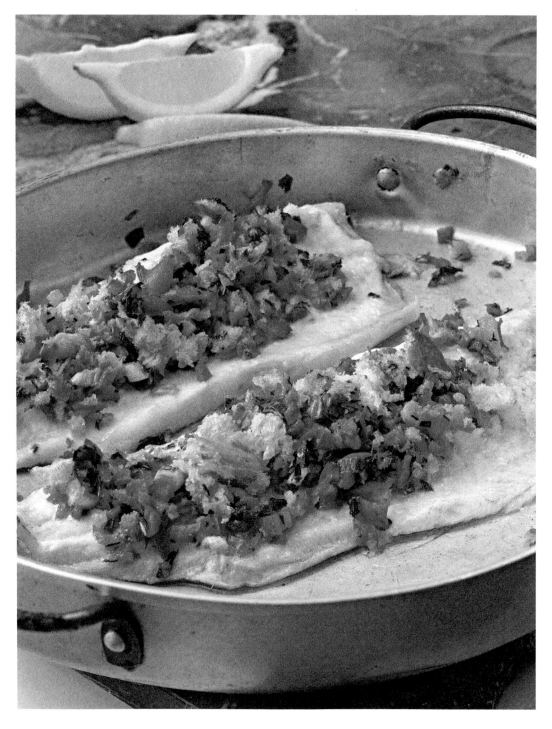

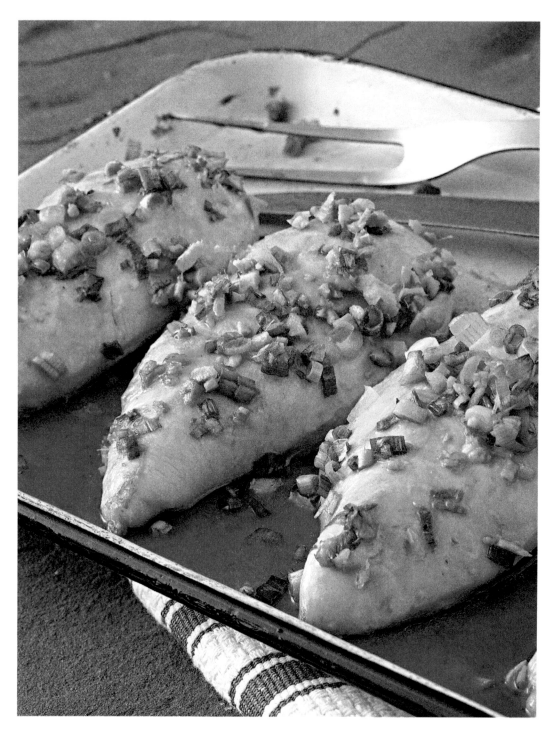

Calming Ginger Chicken

It's no wonder that chicken is the world's primary source of animal protein and a healthy alternative to red meat. It is delicious and can be prepared in a variety of ways, with a wide range of herbs and spices. Chicken is loaded with B vitamins and is a good source of selenium, an important antioxidant that's beneficial to thyroid metabolism and immune function.

INGREDIENTS

2 tablespoons (28 ml) low-sodium
 soy sauce
1 tablespoon (15 ml) sesame oil
3 scallions, thinly sliced
1 teaspoon grated lemon zest
2 teaspoons fresh lemon juice
¼ cup (24 g) minced fresh ginger
4 chicken breasts

Yield: 4 servings

Health Facilitators	Nutrient Density Rating
Protein	Very High
Fat	Low
Carbohydrate	Low
Enzymes	Moderate
Antioxidants	Very High
Fiber	Low

Preheat oven to 350°F (180°C, or gas mark 4). In a small bowl, stir together soy sauce, sesame oil, scallions, lemon zest, lemon juice, and fresh ginger. Place chicken in a single layer in an ovenproof baking dish. Spoon soy-ginger mixture over chicken. Place dish in oven and cook for 25 to 30 minutes. When chicken is done, remove from baking dish and keep warm. Pour soy-ginger dressing from pan into a small bowl and serve on top of chicken.

Did You Know?

For more than 2,000 years, ginger's health benefits have been touted for treating problems such as rheumatism, arthritis, blood disorders, coughing, bloating, heartburn, and digestive upset. Ginger is also known for its calming effects, as well as its characteristic taste and fragrance.

Tasty Tofu Satay with Peanut Sauce

The peanut sauce in this dish packs a serious nutritional punch, due to the fact that peanuts are loaded with enough antioxidants to rival apples, carrots, and beets. Peanuts are also good sources of vitamin E, niacin, folate, and proteins, making this a particularly balanced dish.

INGREDIENTS
1½ pounds (680 g) firm tofu
4 to 8 romaine lettuce leaves
4 tablespoons (4 g) chopped fresh parsley

For marinade
4 tablespoons (65 g) peanut butter, smooth or chunky (no sugar added)
2 tablespoons (28 ml) low-sodium tamari soy sauce
2 tablespoons (28 ml) fresh lime juice
1 tablespoon (6 g) fresh ginger, peeled and finely minced
2 garlic cloves, peeled and minced
1 tablespoon (4 g) chopped fresh cilantro
Dash cayenne pepper

Eight 8-inch (20-cm) bamboo skewers, soaked in water for 15 minutes to prevent burning

Yield: 4 servings

To prepare tofu, drain and cut into 1½-inch (3.75-cm) pieces; set aside. In a blender or food processor, blend marinade ingredients until smooth. Add 1 to 2 teaspoons hot water, if needed, to thin marinade. Taste, and adjust seasonings.

Mix tofu with marinade. Place in container, cover and marinate, refrigerated, for at least 30 minutes, or overnight if possible, mixing occasionally.

Preheat broiler. Thread tofu onto skewers. Arrange skewers on a greased rack with a tinfoil-lined baking sheet underneath. Broil them, turning occasionally, until evenly browned, about 10 minutes per side. Brush with extra marinade before serving. Serve on a bed of romaine lettuce and garnish with chopped parsley.

Did You Know?
Tofu—also known as soy bean curd—has been called the perfect food. It is high in protein and is a good source of calcium and vitamin E.

Health Facilitators	Nutrient Density Rating
Protein	Very High
Fat	Low
Carbohydrate	High
Enzymes	High
Antioxidants	Very High
Fiber	High

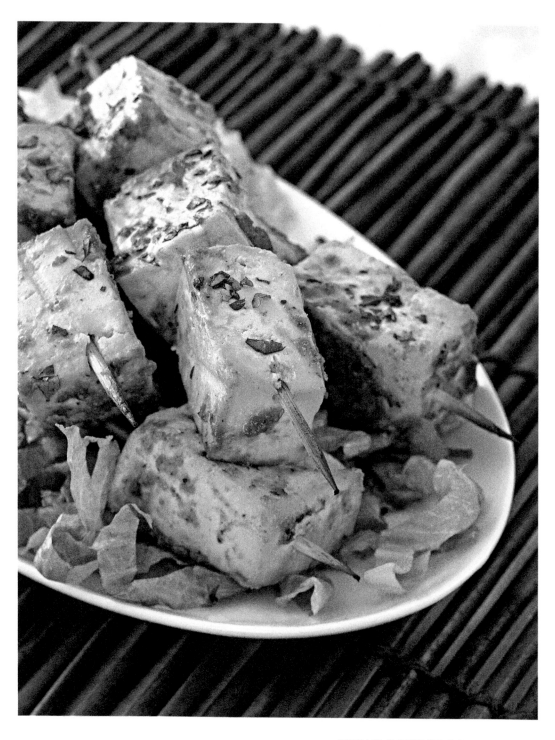

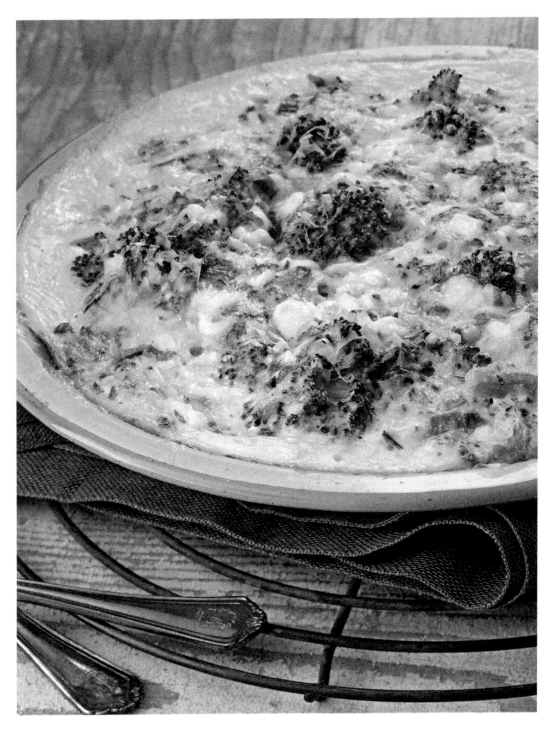

Sunny Broccoli Cheese Pie

Broccoli is well known for its numerous phytochemicals and antioxidants such as beta-carotene and vitamin C, plus it is a super-rich source of calcium and other important minerals. This dish is also high in fiber, and loaded with protein from the three cheeses. You'll want to skip this recipe if your allergic to dairy products.

INGREDIENTS

2 tablespoons (28 g) unsalted butter
²/₃ cup (75 g) thinly sliced scallions
2½ cups (175 g) broccoli florets
   (or 20 ounces [560 g] frozen broccoli
   thawed and drained), chopped and
   lightly steamed
1½ (340 g) cups whole-milk cottage
   cheese or whole-milk ricotta cheese
3 eggs, beaten
2 ounces (8 g) crumbled Gorgonzola
   or other blue-veined cheese
¼ cup (4 g) minced fresh parsley
2 tablespoons (5 g) slivered fresh basil
3 tablespoons (24 g) regular or
   gluten-free flour
Freshly ground black pepper to taste
Dash cayenne pepper
2 tablespoons (10 g) grated
   Parmesan cheese
3 tablespoons (27 g) sunflower seeds

Yield: 6 servings

Preheat oven to 350°F (180°C, or gas mark 4). In a large frying-pan or skillet, melt butter over medium-high heat. When butter is hot and bubbling, reduce heat to medium. Add scallions and sauté until softened, about 3 minutes. In a large bowl, using a fork, mix the sautéed scallions, broccoli, cottage or ricotta cheese, eggs, Gorgonzola cheese, parsley, basil, flour, black pepper, and cayenne pepper.

Pour filling into a buttered 9-inch square (23-cm) baking pan or soufflé dish. Top with Parmesan cheese and bake until puffed and golden brown, 30 to 35 minutes. Broil for 1 minute to brown top. Let cool 5 minutes before slicing. Serve sprinkled with sunflower seeds and garnished with fresh parsley.

Did You Know?

Sunflower seeds are an excellent source of vitamin E, the body's primary fat-soluble antioxidant, and they have significant anti-inflammatory effects, which makes them particularly helpful with arthritis and joint problems.

Health Facilitators	Nutrient Density Rating
Protein	Very High
Fat	Moderate
Carbohydrate	Very High
Enzymes	Very High
Antioxidants	Very High
Fiber	Very High

Zucchini and Mushroom Quiche

Zucchini is an excellent source of the antioxidants vitamin C, beta-carotene, and lutein, which promote eye health and are anti-inflammatory. Mushrooms are probiotic and help the body restore balance and regain strength. If your allergic to dairy products you might want to skip this recipe, or substitute with goat or sheep cheese.

INGREDIENTS

For rice crust

2½ cups (412 g) cooked brown rice
2 tablespoons (28 g) unsalted butter, melted
1 egg, beaten
1 tablespoon (8 g) regular or gluten-free flour
1 tablespoon (4 g) minced fresh parsley
2 tablespoons (12 g) minced scallions
Dash of ground black pepper

For filling

2 tablespoons (28 g) unsalted butter
1 small red onion, diced
1 pound (454 g) thinly sliced zucchini
2 cups (140 g) sliced reishi or shiitake mushrooms
1 cup (230 g) whole-milk cottage cheese or whole-milk ricotta cheese
3 eggs
2 tablespoons (28 ml) heavy cream
2 tablespoons (10 g) grated Parmesan cheese
2 tablespoons (5 g) slivered fresh basil, or 1 teaspoon dried basil
Freshly ground black pepper, to taste
2 tablespoons (8 g) fresh chopped parsley to garnish

Yield: 6 servings

To make the crust: Preheat oven to 350°F (180°C, or gas mark 4). Lightly butter a 9-inch (23-cm) pie pan. In a medium bowl, using a fork, combine all crust ingredients. Mix well. Gently pat into pie pan, pressing against the edges and bottom of pan. Bake for 20 minutes, until evenly browned. Let cool.

To make the filling: Preheat oven to 325°F (170°C, or gas mark 3). In a large frying pan or skillet, melt butter over medium-high heat. When butter is hot and bubbling, add onion, and sauté until softened, about 3 minutes. Add zucchini and mushrooms, and sauté until tender, about 7 minutes. Drain well and set aside.

In a medium bowl, combine cottage or ricotta cheese, eggs, cream, Parmesan cheese, basil, and pepper. Add sautéed vegetables and pour into prepared rice crust. Bake until filling is browned and set, about 30 minutes. Garnish with fresh parsley.

Health Facilitators	Nutrient Density Rating
Protein	Very High
Fat	Moderate
Carbohydrate	Very High
Enzymes	High
Antioxidants	Very High
Fiber	Very High

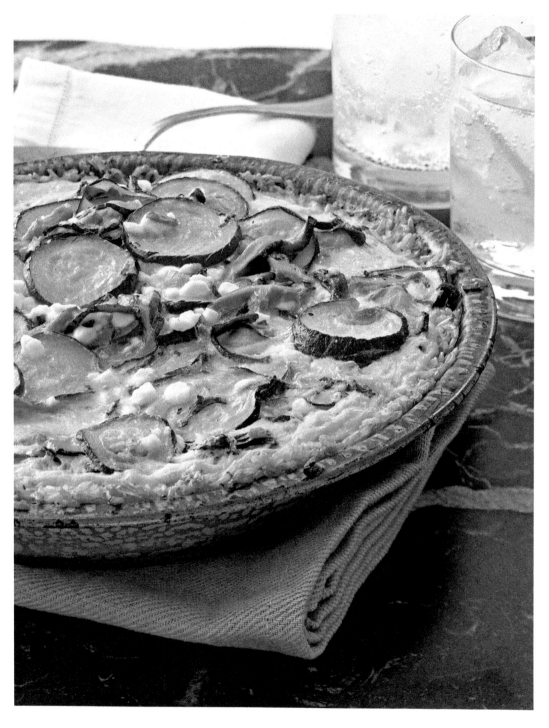

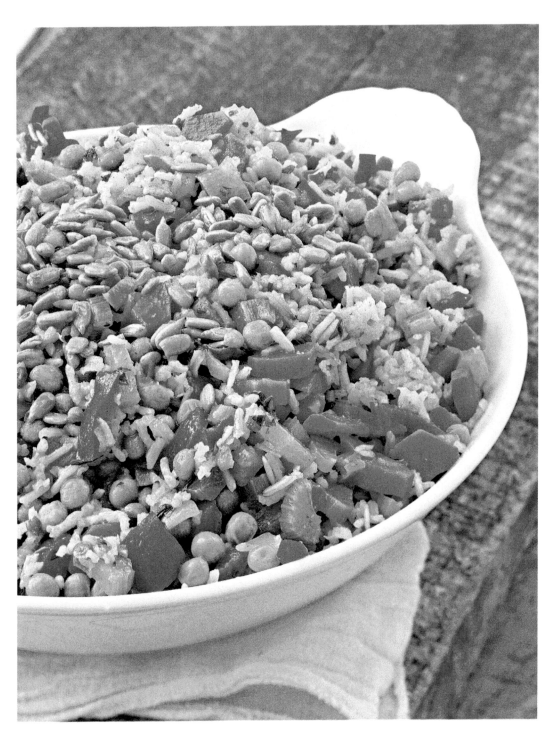

Powerful Pilaf

Whole-grain brown rice is a rich source of phytochemicals and antioxidants to boost your immune system. Its mix of B vitamins, magnesium, iron, fiber, and vitamin E makes it even more powerful. Mushrooms, garlic, celery, herbs, and spices combine here to provide you with a full array of nourishing nutrients that fortify your immune system.

INGREDIENTS

2 tablespoons (28 ml) pure-pressed extra-virgin olive oil
1 medium onion, finely diced
4 carrots, diced
4 stalks celery, diced
1¼ cups (152 g) whole-grain brown rice
2 red or green bell peppers, diced
½ cup (75 g) fresh or (65 g) frozen green peas
1 cup (70 g) sliced shiitake or reishi mushrooms
2½ cups (588 ml) vegetable (or chicken) stock or filtered water
1½ teaspoons chopped fresh thyme, or ½ teaspoon dried thyme
2 tablespoons (8 g) chopped fresh parsley
1 teaspoon chili powder
1 teaspoon dried oregano
1 teaspoon ground cumin
2 or 3 cloves garlic, peeled and finely chopped
Freshly ground black pepper and Himalayan crystal salt to taste
1 to 2 tablespoons (9 to 18 g) sunflower seeds
4 to 8 romaine lettuce leaves

Yield: 4 servings

Preheat oven to 350°F (180°C, or gas mark 4). In a large saucepan, heat the oil and sauté the onion, carrots, and celery over low heat for about 8 minutes. Add the rice and continue to cook until rice is lightly browned. Remove from heat, add the remaining ingredients, and mix well. Transfer the mixture to a 1-quart (946-ml) casserole dish and bake, covered, for 30 to 40 minutes, until liquid is absorbed and rice is soft. Garnish with sunflower seeds. Serve on a bed of romaine lettuce or with a leafy green salad.

Health Facilitators	Nutrient Density Rating
Protein	Very High
Fat	Low
Carbohydrate	Very High
Enzymes	High
Antioxidants	Very High
Fiber	Very High

Mighty Mushroom Risotto

Shiitake mushrooms stimulate the immune system, have anti-cancer properties, and help fight infections. They also treat nutritional deficiencies and boost liver function. The rice provides high fiber, B vitamins, and protein. If your allergic to dairy products, it's okay to leave them out.

INGREDIENTS

1 cup (135 g) pine nuts
3 tablespoons (45 ml) pure-pressed extra-virgin olive oil
2 garlic cloves, peeled and minced
1 small onion, diced
½ pound (225 g) thinly sliced shiitake mushrooms
½ cup (28 g) sun-dried tomatoes packed in oil, drained and slivered
1½ cups (285 g) whole-grain brown rice, rinsed and drained
5 cups (1.2 L) vegetable stock
¼ cup (10 g) slivered fresh basil, or 2 teaspoons dried basil
1 cup (120 g) crumbled Gorgonzola cheese (optional)
2 teaspoons grated lemon zest
¼ cup (60 ml) organic cream
Freshly ground black pepper to taste
½ cup (30 g) fresh parsley, chopped

Yield: 8 servings

Health Facilitators	Nutrient Density Rating
Protein	Very High
Fat	Moderate
Carbohydrate	High
Enzymes	High
Antioxidants	Very High
Fiber	Very High

Put pine nuts in an ungreased skillet over medium-high heat. Stir nuts or shake pan almost constantly, until pine nuts are evenly browned and toasted. Remove from pan immediately and set aside.

In a large saucepan, heat oil over medium-high heat. When oil is hot, add garlic, onion, and mushrooms and sauté until softened, about 5 minutes. Add sun-dried tomatoes and long-grain brown rice, and stir gently to thoroughly coat grains of rice with oil.

In another saucepan, bring stock to a boil and reduce heat to low. Ladle 1 cup (235 ml) of simmering stock into rice and stir well. Cook over medium heat, uncovered, stirring constantly until all liquid is absorbed. Add another cup of hot stock and stir constantly until all liquid is absorbed. Continue adding one cup at a time, until all of stock has been absorbed and rice is tender. (This should take 20 to 30 minutes.)

After stock has been added and rice is cooked to your liking, add basil, Gorgonzola cheese, lemon zest, cream, and black pepper. Taste, and adjust seasonings. Sprinkle with pine nuts and garnish with fresh parsley.

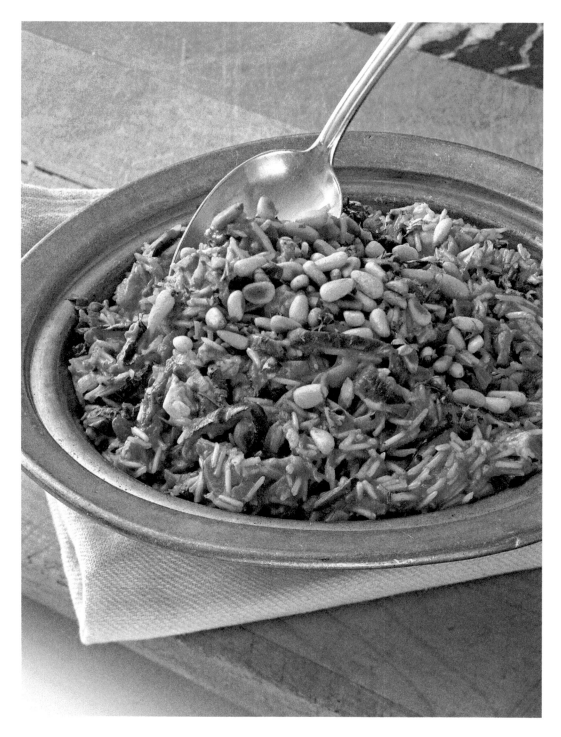

Beneficial Brown Rice

Brown rice is loaded with B vitamins, magnesium, and manganese, and it is one of the world's healthiest foods. It is also a good source of selenium—a mineral known for reducing the risk of colon cancer—and anti-inflammatory nutrients, which make it a good staple for people with muscle, joint, or rheumatic conditions.

INGREDIENTS

2 tablespoons (28 g) unsalted butter
2 tablespoons (28 ml) pure-pressed
  extra-virgin olive oil
1 green bell pepper, diced
1 medium red onion, diced
2 garlic cloves, peeled and minced
2 celery stalks, diced
1 teaspoon ground cumin
1 teaspoon dried oregano
1½ cups (285 g) whole-grain brown rice,
  rinsed and drained
1½ cups (270 g) diced tomato
3 cups (705 ml) vegetable stock
  or filtered water
Freshly ground black pepper to taste
1 cup (150 g) fresh green peas,
  or 1 cup (130 g) frozen and thawed
2 tablespoons (8 g) minced fresh parsley
¼ cup (25 g) chopped black or green
  olives
4 tablespoons (20 g) grated Romano or
  Parmesan cheese (optional)
1 head of romaine lettuce, washed
  and drained

Yield: 8 servings

In a medium saucepan with a tight-fitting lid, heat butter and oil over medium-high heat. When hot, add green pepper, onion, garlic, celery, cumin, and oregano. Sauté until softened, about 5 minutes. Add rice, and sauté until coated with butter and oil, about 2 minutes. Add tomatoes, stock or water, and black pepper, and stir well.

Bring to a boil. Cover tightly, and reduce heat to simmer. Simmer for 45 minutes, until all liquid is absorbed. Remove from heat and let sit, covered and undisturbed, for 10 minutes. Remove lid and fluff rice with a fork. Stir in peas, parsley and olives. Taste, and adjust seasonings. Sprinkle with grated cheese. Serve on a bed of romaine lettuce leaves or with a green leafy salad.

Health Facilitators	Nutrient Density Rating
Protein	Very High
Fat	Moderate
Carbohydrate	Very High
Enzymes	High
Antioxidants	Very High
Fiber	Very High

Lively Black Bean Chili

Black beans are a wonderful source of dietary fiber, which helps keep blood sugar levels stable after a meal. They are rich in antioxidants and are a wise choice for people with low energy or people who have hypoglycemia. When black beans are prepared with whole grains such as barley or wild rice, they provide a high-quality source of protein. Use goat's or sheep's cheese if your allergic to cow products.

INGREDIENTS

For chili

1 pound (454 g) dried black beans, rinsed, and soaked overnight
7 cups (1.6 L) filtered water
2 tablespoons (28 ml) pure-pressed extra-virgin olive oil
1 medium onion, chopped
2 garlic cloves, peeled and minced
1 small fresh jalapeño pepper, diced
1 green bell pepper, chopped
2 teaspoons ground cumin
2 teaspoons dried oregano
1 teaspoon chili powder
2 bay leaves
½ teaspoon red pepper flakes
28 ounces (828 ml) canned tomatoes, chopped (liquid reserved)
2 tablespoons (8 g) fresh cilantro, chopped
Freshly ground black pepper to taste
1 tablespoon (15 ml) fresh lime juice

For topping

2 cups (240 g) grated cheddar cheese (optional)
1 cup (235 ml) whole-milk sour cream (optional)
½ bunch parsley for garnish

Yield: 8 servings

Drain black beans. In a heavy-bottomed soup pot, cover beans with water and bring to a boil. Reduce heat to medium and cook, uncovered, until beans are tender, about 45 minutes to 1 hour, skimming any foam that collects on the surface.

In a large frying pan or skillet, heat oil over medium-high heat. When oil is hot, add onion, garlic, jalapeño pepper, bell pepper, cumin, oregano, and chili powder. Sauté until vegetables are softened and tender, about 10 minutes.

Add sautéed vegetables, bay leaves, red pepper flakes, tomatoes and their juice, cilantro, and black pepper to cooked beans. Cook over low heat for 30 minutes. Add lime juice. Taste, and adjust seasonings. Ladle into bowls and top with grated cheese and a spoonful of sour cream. Garnish generously with fresh parsley.

Health Facilitators	Nutrient Density Rating
Protein	High
Fat	Low
Carbohydrate	High
Enzymes	Moderate
Antioxidants	Very High
Fiber	Very High

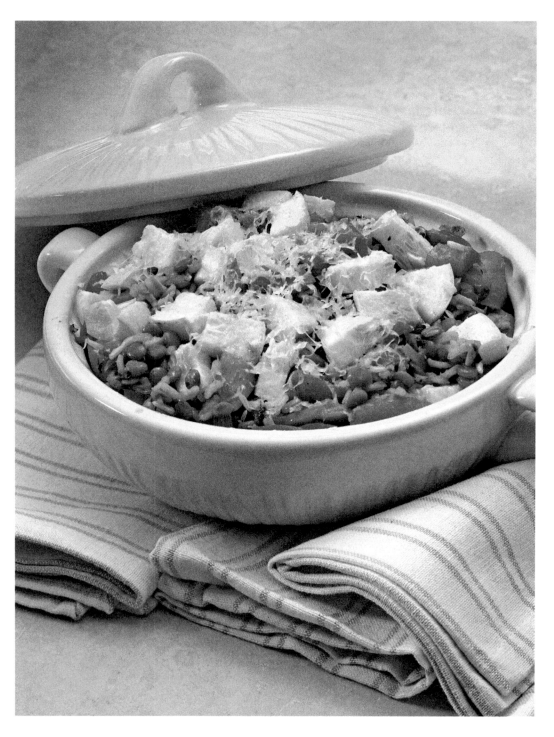

Lusty Lentil Casserole

Lentils are nutritious, flavorful, and a good source of protein, calcium, B vitamins, and iron. High in fiber, this tiny nutritional giant fills you up—not out. The herbs and vegetables add not only to the fresh taste of this casserole but also increase its quotient of nutrients and phytochemicals.

INGREDIENTS

1 cup (190 g) whole-grain brown rice
6 cups (1.4 L) vegetable stock
2 cloves garlic, peeled and minced
1 tablespoon (2.5 g) freshly chopped basil
2 tablespoons (28 ml) pure-pressed extra-virgin olive oil
2 cups (384 g) lentils
12 medium carrots, sliced into small angled chunks (rotate the carrot ¼ turn after each cut)
2 cups (240 g) diced celery
1 small onion, diced
Himalayan crystal salt and freshly ground black pepper to taste
4 tablespoons (15 g) chopped fresh parsley
½ cup (70 g) each of selected vegetables, such as cauliflower, yellow squash, and red peppers
4 tablespoons (20 g) grated Romano or Parmesan cheese
1 head of romaine lettuce or mixed greens

Yield: 8 servings

Preheat oven to 325°F (170°C, or gas mark 3). Place rice, vegetable stock, garlic, basil, and olive oil in a large pot. Rinse and pick over the lentils. Add lentils, carrots, celery, and onion to pot. Bring to a boil, stir once, cover, reduce heat to a simmer, and cook for 45 minutes or until liquid is absorbed and vegetables are tender. Season with salt and pepper to taste, and add the parsley. Transfer contents into a large baking dish and top with selected vegetables. Sprinkle with Romano or Parmesan cheese, and bake in oven for 10 minutes. Serve over a bed of romaine lettuce leaves or with a mixed green salad.

Did You Know?

Brown rice is a high-fiber companion to lentils and is equally loaded with B vitamins, minerals, and protein.

Health Facilitators	Nutrient Density Rating
Protein	Very High
Fat	Low
Carbohydrate	Very High
Enzymes	Moderate
Antioxidants	Very High
Fiber	Very High

Body-Building Barley Casserole

Barley has been used as nourishment and medicine for many centuries. A terrific source of B vitamins, which fight stress and build up the central nervous system, barley is rich in tocotrienols—compounds that act as antioxidants and reduce LDL-cholesterol (a risk factor in cardiovascular disease). Immune-boosting shiitake or reishi mushrooms add to the flavor and nutritional benefits of this delicious dish. Use quinoa or other gluten-free grains if preferred.

INGREDIENTS

3 tablespoons (45 g) unsalted butter
1 to 2 cloves garlic, peeled and minced
1 small onion, chopped
2 cups (140 g) sliced shiitake
  or reishi mushrooms
1 cup (200 g) pearl barley,
  rinsed and drained
3 cups (705 ml) vegetable stock
  or filtered water
Freshly ground black pepper
  and Himalayan crystal salt to taste
1 head of romaine lettuce
2 tablespoons (8 g) fresh chopped parsley
2 tablespoons (10 g) grated Romano
  or Parmesan cheese (optional)

Yield: 4 servings

In a large saucepan with a tight-fitting lid, melt butter over medium-high heat. When butter is hot and bubbling, add garlic and onion and sauté until softened, about 5 minutes. Add mushrooms and barley and sauté for 5 minutes. Add stock or water, bring to a boil, cover and reduce heat to low. Simmer for 60 to 70 minutes, or until all liquid has been absorbed and barley is tender. Season to taste with pepper and salt. Serve on a bed of romaine lettuce, garnish with chopped parsley, and sprinkle with Romano or Parmesan cheese.

Health Facilitators	Nutrient Density Rating
Protein	High
Fat	Low
Carbohydrate	High
Enzymes	High
Antioxidants	Very High
Fiber	Very High

Complete Quinoa with Spinach

Quinoa (pronounced keen-wah), which the Incas referred to as the "mother grain," is one of nature's most complete foods and has a higher protein content than any other grain. The amino acid composition in quinoa is near perfect. The World Health Organization has judged the protein in quinoa to be as complete as that in milk. In addition, quinoa contains more iron than most grains, and it is a good source of calcium, phosphorus, and folate.

INGREDIENTS

2 cups (475 ml) vegetable stock
  or filtered water
1 cup (185 g) quinoa, rinsed and drained
4 cups (120 g) fresh spinach
2 tablespoons (28 ml) pure-pressed
  extra-virgin olive oil
2 garlic cloves, peeled and minced
½ cup (80 g) diced onion
1 cup (180 g) chopped tomatoes
¼ cup (10 g) slivered fresh basil,
  or 2 teaspoons dried basil
1 teaspoon grated lemon zest
½ cup (75 g) crumbled feta cheese
Freshly ground black pepper
  and Himalayan crystal salt, to taste
4 tablespoons (15 g) chopped fresh
  parsley

Yield: 8 servings

In a medium saucepan with a tight-fitting lid, bring stock or water to a boil. Add quinoa and return to a boil. Cover, reduce heat to low, and simmer for 15 minutes or until all liquid has been absorbed. Remove from heat and let sit, covered and undisturbed, for 10 minutes. Set aside.

Wash spinach well, removing stems. With water still clinging to leaves, place in a medium saucepan with a tight-fitting lid. Turn heat to medium-high, and steam until leaves are wilted, about 2 to 3 minutes. Drain in a colander, pressing out all liquid with the back of a wooden spoon. Chop coarsely and set aside.

In a large frying pan or skillet, heat oil over medium-high heat. When oil is hot, add garlic and onion and sauté until softened, about 5 minutes. Add tomatoes and cook for 5 minutes. Add spinach, basil, prepared quinoa, lemon zest, feta cheese, salt, and black pepper. Mix well and cook until heated through. Taste, and adjust seasonings. Garnish with chopped parsley and serve.

Health Facilitators	Nutrient Density Rating
Protein	Very High
Fat	Low
Carbohydrate	Very High
Enzymes	High
Antioxidants	Very High
Fiber	Very High

Stimulating Stir-Fried Vegetables

Whether you choose to add tempeh or tofu to this nourishing dish, you can't go wrong health-wise. Tempeh boosts immune system function, is high in fiber and phytochemicals, and is an excellent source of protein. Tofu is high in protein, as well as calcium and vitamin E. Ginger has long been celebrated for its healing powers, but did you know that ginger has an effect on blood clots that is similar to aspirin? (Only healthier, of course.)

INGREDIENTS

8 ounces (225 g) tofu or tempeh, cut into ½-inch (1.3 cm) cubes
1 cup (70 g) fresh (or reconstituted dried) shiitake mushrooms
1 to 2 tablespoons (15 to 28 ml) coconut oil
1 large onion, chopped
1 cup (235 ml) vegetable stock
2 carrots, sliced on diagonal
1 cup (70 g) broccoli florets
½ cup (62 g) water chestnuts, sliced
1 cup (50 g) bean sprouts
1 clove garlic, minced
2 tablespoons (16 g) grated fresh ginger
Tamari or soy sauce to taste
3 tablespoons (45 ml) toasted sesame oil
Cayenne pepper to taste

Yield: 6 servings

If using tempeh, bake or steam for 10 minutes before cutting into cubes. Remove stems from shiitake mushrooms and reserve to make stock. Slice mushrooms.

In a wok or large skillet, add coconut oil and sauté onion over medium flame until it starts to release

its juice. Add ½ cup (120 ml) of stock and bring to a rapid boil over a high flame. Add shiitake mushrooms, cover, and simmer for 5 minutes. Add carrots, and sauté for a few minutes, adding stock if necessary. Add tofu or tempeh, broccoli, water chestnuts, bean sprouts, and garlic. Sauté for a few minutes, or until broccoli is bright green. Add the fresh grated ginger to vegetables. Stir and cook a minute longer. Remove from heat, season with tamari or soy sauce, toasted sesame oil, and cayenne pepper.

Did You Know?

Water chestnuts are a delicacy in Asian cultures and are rich in potassium and high in fiber.

Health Facilitators	Nutrient Density Rating
Protein	Very High
Fat	Low
Carbohydrate	High
Enzymes	High
Antioxidants	Very High
Fiber	Very High

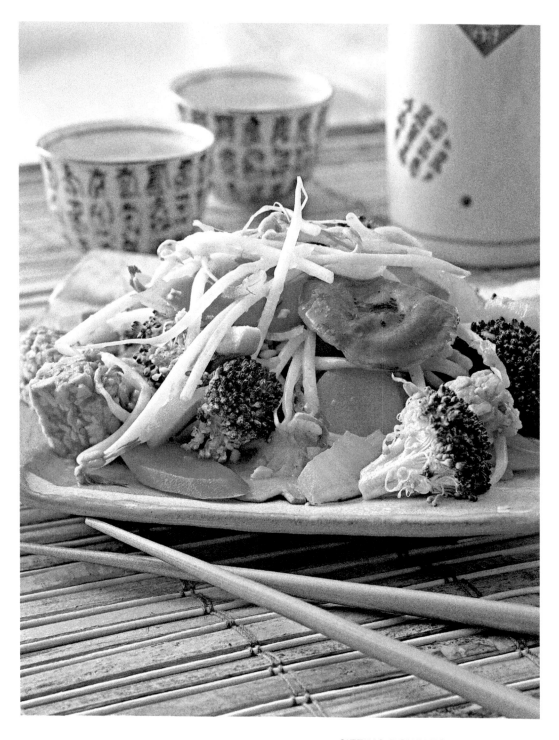

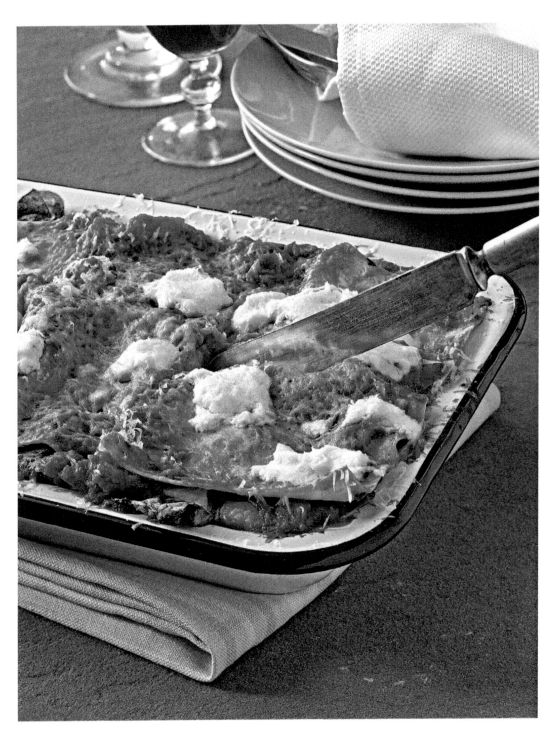

Vegetarian Vitality Lasagna

When you're lacking oomph or zip, and your vitality just isn't what you'd like, you need to re-energize by choosing the right fuel for your body. That's where this dish comes in. A vegetarian lasagna, it is loaded with phytonutrients, antioxidants, enzymes, and fiber, as well as a healthy balance of protein, fats, and carbohydrates. Enjoy its many benefits and get ready to recharge! Use gluten-free pasta if preferred, and goat's or sheep's cheese if allergic to cow products.

INGREDIENTS

2 tablespoons (28 ml) pure-pressed
   extra-virgin olive oil
1 small onion, finely chopped
1 to 2 garlic cloves,
   peeled and finely chopped
1 cup (160 g) minced shallots
1 small carrot, finely chopped
1 stalk celery, finely chopped
4 cups (120 g) fresh spinach, chopped
1 teaspoon ground nutmeg
12 lasagna noodles, slightly cooked
   (if pre-cooking is required)
6 cups (1470 g) tomato sauce
2 cups (200 g) cooked beans
   (kidney, red, black, or white)
3 to 4 tablespoons (27 to 36 g)
   raw sunflower seeds
1 cup (250 g) ricotta cheese,
   or 1 cup tofu (250 g) mashed
   with 1 tablespoon (15 ml) light miso
Himalayan crystal salt and freshly ground
   black pepper to taste
1 cup (100 g) finely grated
   Parmesan cheese

Yield: 6 servings

Preheat oven to 350°F (180°C, or gas mark 4). Heat the oil in skillet and sauté the onions, garlic, and shallots until transparent. Add carrot and celery and cook for 5 to 10 minutes. Combine with spinach and nutmeg.

In a large baking dish, alternate layers of lasagna noodles, tomato sauce, beans, sunflower seeds, spinach mixture, and ricotta or tofu, until ingredients are used up; finish with tomato sauce and ricotta cheese. Season with salt and pepper. Sprinkle with Parmesan cheese. Cover and bake for 20 to 30 minutes. Serve with a leafy green salad.

Health Facilitators	Nutrient Density Rating
Protein	Very High
Fat	Moderate
Carbohydrate	Very High
Enzymes	Moderate
Antioxidants	Very High
Fiber	Very High

Sumptuous Summer Squash Stir-Fry

An excellent source of manganese and vitamin C, summer squash is also a very good source of magnesium, vitamin A (most notably through its concentration of carotenoids, including beta-carotene), fiber, potassium, folate, riboflavin, and phosphorus. Many of these nutrients have been shown to help prevent heart disease and stroke, high blood pressure, inflammation, and cancer.

INGREDIENTS
1 tablespoon (15 ml) pure-pressed extra-virgin olive oil
1 cup (200 g) diced ripe tomatoes
3 cups (340 g) mixed summer squash (zucchini, yellow squash, crook neck, or other) cut into 1-inch (2.5-cm) cubes
1 garlic clove, peeled and minced
1 teaspoon tamari
1 cup (250 g) cubed tofu (optional)
2 tablespoons (18 g) raw sunflower seeds
2 tablespoons (8 g) chopped fresh parsley
Freshly ground black pepper and Himalayan crystal salt to taste

Yield: 4 servings

Heat oil in a medium-size skillet. Add vegetables and sauté until tender. Add garlic and tamari, stirring to coat vegetables well. Continue to cook 5 more minutes. Add tofu, if desired. Add freshly ground black pepper and salt to taste. Sprinkle with sunflower seeds and chopped parsley.

Health Facilitators	Nutrient Density Rating
Protein	Low
Fat	Low
Carbohydrate	Very High
Enzymes	High
Antioxidants	Very High
Fiber	Very High

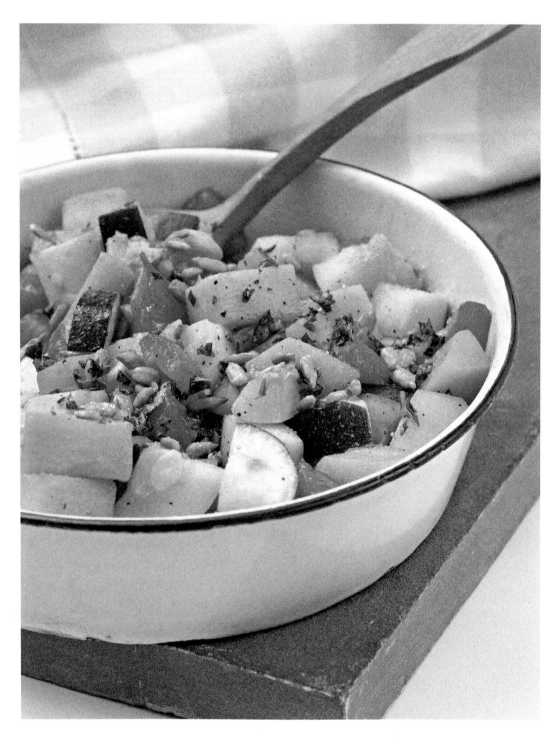

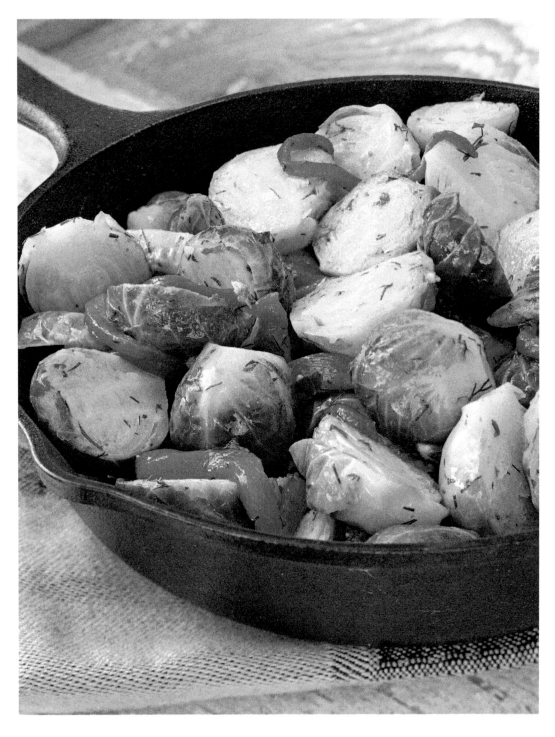

Cleansing Red Peppers and Brussels Sprouts

Brussels sprouts enhance the activity of the body's natural defense systems to protect against disease, including cancer. They contain substances known to stimulate the liver to produce enzymes that detoxify chemicals and carcinogens, making this vegetable particularly cleansing and nourishing to the body. They also happen to be loaded with phytonutrients, vitamins, and minerals.

INGREDIENTS

2 red bell peppers, cut in half
½ tablespoon (7.5 ml) pure-pressed extra-virgin olive oil
1½ pounds (3 cups or 680 g) cooked brussels sprouts
1 clove garlic, peeled and minced
Himalayan crystal salt to taste
Freshly ground black pepper to taste
1 tablespoon (4 g) minced fresh dill

Yield: 8 servings

Preheat oven to 350°F (180°C, or gas mark 4). Place peppers on a cookie sheet and brush with oil. Bake for 30 minutes. Remove peppers from oven, let cool, then peel and seed. Cut peppers into ¼-inch (6-mm) strips. Place cooked brussels sprouts in a glass or ceramic baking dish or in a cast-iron skillet. Stir in pepper strips. Add garlic, salt, and pepper and toss to mix well. Bake uncovered for 10 minutes and garnish with fresh dill.

Did You Know?

Red peppers are an excellent source of vitamins A and C. They contain high antioxidant levels, and they have been linked to a reduced risk of heart disease and cancer.

Health Facilitators	Nutrient Density Rating
Protein	Low
Fat	Low
Carbohydrate	Very High
Enzymes	High
Antioxidants	Very High
Fiber	Very High

Super Spinach with Mushrooms

Spinach has been called a superfood because of its rich nutrient content and low calorie count. It has a family of phytonutrients that include carotenoids, lutein, beta-carotene, and quercetin. Shiitake mushrooms have been used for centuries by the Chinese and Japanese to treat colds and flu. They appear to stimulate the immune system, help fight infection, and demonstrate anti-tumor activity.

INGREDIENTS

8 cups (180 g) fresh spinach
2 garlic cloves, peeled and finely
chopped
Himalayan crystal salt to taste
Freshly ground black pepper to taste
4 tablespoons (55 g) unsalted butter
2 tablespoons (20 g) chopped red onion
2 cups (140 g) thinly sliced shiitake
or reishi mushrooms
1 teaspoon grated lemon zest
1 tablespoon (8 g) whole-wheat or
gluten-free flour
1 teaspoon prepared Dijon mustard
½ cup (120 ml) all-dairy heavy cream,
heated to simmering

Yield: 4 servings

Wash spinach well and remove stems. With water still clinging to leaves, place spinach in a medium saucepan with a tight-fitting lid. Add garlic, salt, and pepper. Turn heat to medium-high and steam until leaves are wilted, 2 to 3 minutes. Drain in a colander, pressing out all liquid with the back of a wooden spoon. Chop fine and set aside.

In a large frying pan or skillet, melt 2 tablespoons (28 g) butter over medium-high heat. When butter is hot and bubbling, add onion and mushrooms, and sauté until softened, about 5 minutes. Add lemon zest, and season to taste with additional black pepper. Remove from pan and set aside.

Melt remaining 2 tablespoons (28 g) butter in same skillet. Add flour and mustard, and cook for 2 minutes over medium heat, stirring constantly. Whisk in the hot cream and stir until smooth and thickened. Add chopped spinach, onion, and mushrooms, and stir well. Cook until heated through. Taste, and adjust seasonings.

Health Facilitators	Nutrient Density Rating
Protein	Moderate
Fat	Moderate
Carbohydrate	Very High
Enzymes	High
Antioxidants	Very High
Fiber	Very High

Jolly Green Beans with Sesame Mayonnaise

Green beans are loaded with nutrients and are an excellent source of protein, fiber, and complex carbohydrates that are low on the glycemic index. They are a rich source of vitamin A, vitamin C, folic acid, and vitamin B6, while providing significant amounts of iron, phosphorus, magnesium, manganese, calcium, and potassium. Combine green beans with sesame seeds and oil for added calcium, magnesium, iron, zinc, B1, and phosphorus.

INGREDIENTS

1 to 2 tablespoons (8 to 16 g)
    sesame seeds
1 pound (454 g) fresh green beans,
    ends trimmed
1/3 cup (75 g) mayonnaise
2 tablespoons (30 g) whole-milk
    sour cream
2 teaspoons fresh lime juice
½ to 1 teaspoon sesame oil
Freshly ground black pepper to taste
Himalayan crystal salt to taste
Dash cayenne pepper

Yield: 4 servings

Place sesame seeds in an ungreased skillet over medium-high heat. Shake pan or stir seeds almost constantly, until seeds are evenly browned and toasted and begin to pop. Remove from pan immediately and set aside.

Cook green beans in boiling water until just tender, about 5 minutes. Drain well and arrange on a serving platter.

In a small bowl, using a fork, mix mayonnaise, sour cream, lime juice, sesame oil, black pepper, salt, and cayenne pepper until well blended. Taste, and adjust seasonings. Pour sauce over green beans and sprinkle with sesame seeds. Serve at room temperature.

Health Facilitators	Nutrient Density Rating
Protein	High
Fat	Low
Carbohydrate	Very High
Enzymes	High
Antioxidants	Very High
Fiber	Very High

Sturdy Spinach and Feta-Filled Tomatoes

We all know that Popeye got super strong by eating spinach, but you may be surprised to learn that he was also protecting himself against osteoporosis, colon cancer, arthritis, and heart disease. Researchers have identified more than thirteen different phytonutrient compounds in spinach. Why are they so important? Because phytonutrients contain high levels of powerful antioxidants, which your body needs to protect it and stay healthy.

INGREDIENTS

2 large firm tomatoes
4 cups (120 g) fresh spinach
2 tablespoons (28 g) unsalted butter
1 to 2 garlic cloves, peeled and minced
1 small red onion, diced
½ cup (75 g) feta cheese
½ cup (25 g fresh or 60 g dried) whole-grain bread crumbs
1 tablespoon (11 g) prepared Dijon mustard
2 tablespoons (5 g) slivered fresh basil, or 2 teaspoons dried basil
1 egg, beaten
Himalayan crystal salt and freshly ground black pepper to taste
Dash cayenne pepper
1 tablespoon (5 g) grated Parmesan cheese
4 raw walnut halves

Yield: 4 servings

Preheat oven to 350°F (180°C, or gas mark 4). Cut tomatoes in half crosswise and scoop out pulp and seeds, leaving shells intact. Wash spinach well, removing stems. With water still clinging to leaves, place in a medium saucepan with a tight-fitting lid. Turn heat to medium-high, and steam until leaves are wilted, 2 to 3 minutes. Drain in a colander, pressing out all liquid with the back of a wooden spoon. Chop coarsely and set aside.

In a small frying pan or skillet, melt butter over medium-high heat. When butter is hot and bubbling, add garlic and onion and sauté until softened, about 5 minutes. Remove from heat and set aside.

In a medium bowl, using a fork, combine prepared spinach, feta cheese, bread crumbs, mustard, basil, egg, salt, black pepper, cayenne pepper, and sautéed onion and garlic. Mix well. Mound some filling into each tomato half. Sprinkle with Parmesan cheese and set on a lightly greased baking sheet. Bake 10 to 15 minutes, or until filling is heated through. Garnish each tomato half with a walnut half.

Health Facilitators	Nutrient Density Rating
Protein	High
Fat	Low
Carbohydrate	Very High
Enzymes	Low
Antioxidants	Very High
Fiber	Very High

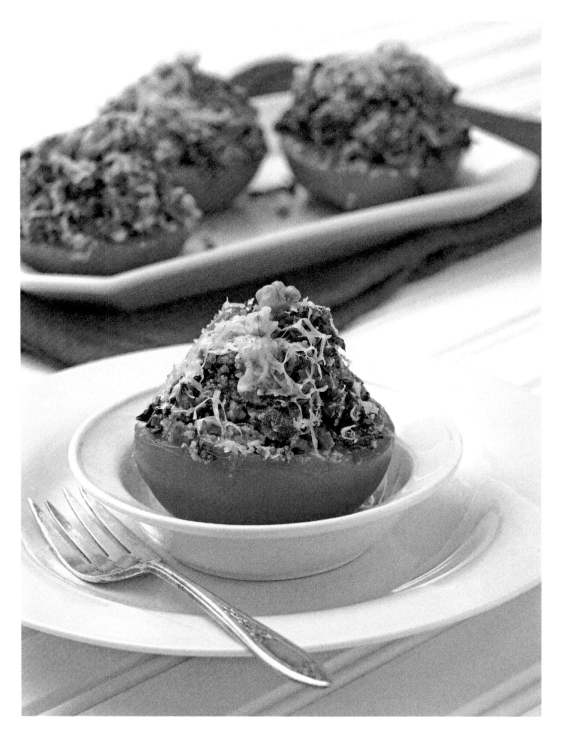

Honeyed Sweet Potatoes

Sweet potatoes are a root vegetable that can be eaten in sweet or savory dishes. They are exceptionally high in vitamin A and a very good source of vitamin C. Both of these powerful antioxidants have anti-inflammatory properties, which can aid in soothing joints, muscles, and arthritis. Sweet potatoes are also a good source of vitamin B6 and are high in fiber.

INGREDIENTS

6 medium sweet potatoes
1 teaspoon butter
½ cup (170 g) honey
1 to 2 teaspoons ground cinnamon
1 to 2 tablespoons (15 to 28 ml) flaxseed oil
1 to 2 tablespoons (4 to 8 g) chopped fresh parsley

Yield: 6 servings

Preheat oven to 350°F (180°C, or gas mark 4). Cook sweet potatoes in boiling salted water until they are just tender. Drain and let cool. Cut potatoes crosswise into ¼-inch (6-mm) slices. Place sliced potatoes in a casserole dish lightly greased with butter. Drizzle with honey, sprinkle with cinnamon, and bake for 35 minutes, basting the sweet potatoes with the honey and cinnamon until they are nicely glazed. Drizzle with flax oil, sprinkle with chopped parsley, and serve immediately.

Health Facilitators	Nutrient Density Rating
Protein	Low
Fat	Low
Carbohydrate	Very High
Enzymes	Low
Antioxidants	Very High
Fiber	Very High

Did You Know?

Sweet potatoes are low on the glycemic index, making them a good choice for stabilizing blood sugar levels.

Potent Potatoes with Vegetable Salsa

Potatoes are the comfort food of choice for many people. They also happen to be a very good source of vitamin C and a good source of vitamin B6, copper, potassium, manganese, and dietary fiber. By combining potatoes with colorful peppers, cilantro, garlic, and tomatoes, this dish delivers even higher levels of free-radical fighters, plus many important vitamins and minerals.

INGREDIENTS

2 Idaho or russet baking potatoes

2 medium sweet potatoes

1 tablespoon (15 ml) pure-pressed extra-virgin olive oil

½ red bell pepper, seeded and diced

½ yellow bell pepper, seeded and diced

½ green bell pepper, seeded and diced

1 medium red onion, diced

1 to 2 cloves garlic, peeled and chopped

4 plum tomatoes, diced

1 teaspoon chopped cilantro

1 tablespoon (15 ml) freshly squeezed lime juice

¼ cup (25 g) grated Parmesan cheese

2 tablespoons (8 g) chopped fresh parsley

Yield: 4 servings

Preheat oven to 400°F (200°C, or gas mark 6). Bake white and sweet potatoes for 50 to 60 minutes, or until soft. Allow to cool slightly and then cut in half. Heat olive oil in a skillet over medium heat and sauté the peppers, onion, and garlic until softened. Add plum tomatoes, cilantro, and lime juice to the pepper mixture. Cook until tomatoes are heated through. Pour salsa over the potato halves, sprinkle with Parmesan cheese, and return them to the oven until cheese is lightly browned, about 5 minutes. Sprinkle with chopped parsley and serve.

Did You Know?

Both sweet potatoes and regular white potatoes contain a potent variety of phytonutrients with antioxidant properties. Among these important health-promoting compounds are carotenoids and flavonoids, which boost the immune system.

Health Facilitators	Nutrient Density Rating
Protein	Moderate
Fat	Low
Carbohydrate	Very High
Enzymes	High
Antioxidants	Very High
Fiber	Very High

Zesty Broccoli with Garlic and Ginger

Broccoli is among the superfoods that contain healthy minerals in abundance. Loaded with magnesium, calcium, and potassium, it is enhanced with the flavors of garlic and ginger. Add it to any cooked grain, meat, fish, or salad. One cup (70 g) of broccoli contains the RDA of vitamin C, an antioxidant that reduces inflammation and builds strong blood vessels.

INGREDIENTS

4 cups (280 g) broccoli florets, cut into quarters
2 tablespoons (30 ml) extra virgin olive oil
2 tablespoons (12 g) finely chopped fresh ginger
2 cloves garlic, finely chopped
2 tablespoons (30 ml) fresh lemon or lime juice

Yield: 4 cups (284 g)

Place the broccoli into a steamer with 2 inches (5 cm) of water. Let steam for 5 to 10 minutes. In a separate bowl, combine the olive oil, ginger, garlic, and lemon juice. Arrange the broccoli in a serving dish and pour the herb mixture on top. Serve hot.

Health Facilitators	Nutrient Density Rating
Protein	Low
Fat	Low
Carbohydrate	High
Enzymes	Low
Antioxidants	Moderate
Fiber	High

Brussels Sprouts with Shiitake and Pine Nuts

The combination of brussels sprouts and shiitake mushrooms makes this dish a medicinal powerhouse that is rich in plant protein, dietary fiber, minerals, and antioxidants that work wonders on your health. You'll love the crunchy texture and creamy combination of the flavors in this delicious side dish that will fill you up without filling you out.

INGREDIENTS

4 cups (352 g) brussels sprouts
4 shiitake mushrooms, soaked in water, drained, and sliced
½ cup (68 g) pine nuts or sunflower seeds
½ teaspoon ground ginger
1 clove garlic, finely chopped
1 cup (235 ml) filtered water
Dash of sea salt or Himalayan salt
Dash of cayenne pepper

Yield: 4 cups (352 g)

Place the brussels sprouts in a steamer and cook for 10 minutes, until tender. In a saucepan, cook the mushrooms, pine nuts, ginger, and garlic in the water until tender. Arrange the brussels sprouts on a serving dish and pour the mushroom mixture on top. Season with salt and cayenne. Serve hot.

Health Facilitators	Nutrient Density Rating
Protein	Low
Fat	Low
Carbohydrate	High
Enzymes	Low
Antioxidants	High
Fiber	High

Colon-Cleansing Cauliflower with Chive Butter

Just three cauliflower florets a day provide 67 percent of your daily vitamin C requirement. Cauliflower also contains folate, a B vitamin we need for cell growth and replication. In addition, cauliflower is an excellent source of fiber, which helps to improve colon health and can prevent cancer. This dish is delicious on it own or served with fish, chicken, brown rice, or other vegetables. Enjoy!

INGREDIENTS

2 heads cauliflower
2 tablespoons (28 g) unsalted butter
¼ cup (12 g) chopped fresh chives
1 teaspoon freshly squeezed lemon juice
2 to 4 tablespoons (8 to 16 g)
   chopped fresh parsley
2 to 4 tablespoons (18 to 36 g) feta
   or (10 to 20 g) grated Parmesan cheese
Freshly ground black pepper
   and Himalayan crystal salt to taste

Yield: 8 servings

Wash cauliflower and break it into florets. Steam until tender, approximately 15 minutes. In a small saucepan, melt butter over low heat and combine with the remaining ingredients. Pour this chive butter over cauliflower florets. Sprinkle with more grated Parmesan cheese and chopped parsley. Serve warm.

Did You Know?

Chives have high levels of vitamin A and C and essential minerals such as potassium, calcium, and folate. They are thought to be mildly antibiotic, which helps boost the immune system.

Health Facilitators	Nutrient Density Rating
Protein	Low
Fat	Low
Carbohydrate	Very High
Enzymes	Moderate
Antioxidants	Very High
Fiber	Very High

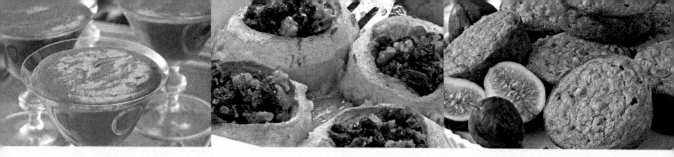

CHAPTER 11

FEEDING YOUR FANCY

Blissful Nut and Seed Balls (RAW)

Nuts are one of the best plant sources of protein. They are rich in fiber, phytonutrients, and antioxidants, such as vitamin E and selenium. Nuts are also high in calcium, magnesium, potassium, and essential oils, such as omega-3 fatty acids. The health benefits of nuts are huge—from preventing heart disease to boosting immunity. Go nuts on this one!

INGREDIENTS
½ cup (130 g) raw almond butter
½ cup (120 g) tahini
1 teaspoon vanilla extract
½ teaspoon cinnamon
½ teaspoon nutmeg
¼ teaspoon fresh ground ginger
¼ cup (25 g) carob powder
¼ cup (35 g) pine nuts or hemp seeds

Yield: 1 dozen

Combine the almond butter, tahini, vanilla extract, cinnamon, nutmeg, and fresh ground ginger in a large mixing bowl. Form into balls and roll in carob powder and pine nuts or hemp seeds.

Did You Know?
Hemp seeds are rich in essential fatty acids and are considered a complete protein food source. You can purchase them online or in health food stores

Health Facilitators	Nutrient Density Rating
Protein	Very High
Fat	Low
Carbohydrate	High
Enzymes	Very High
Antioxidants	Very High
Fiber	Very High

Cathartic Carob Fudge (RAW)

Carob is a delicious alternative to chocolate and does not contain the cholesterol, caffeine, theobromine, or oxalic acid in chocolate. Carob is high in fiber, low in sodium, calcium-rich and has a natural sweetness, which reduces the need for additional sweeteners. Add to this the many benefits of coconuts and apricots, and your waistline and taste buds will thank you for this treat.

INGREDIENTS

1 cup (145 g) raw carob powder
½ cup (45 g) almonds, soaked overnight
   in purified or spring water,
   drained, and chopped
½ cup (120 ml) coconut oil
½ teaspoon vanilla
2 dried apricots, soaked in purified
   or spring water for an hour, and drained

Yield: 20 squares

Blend all ingredients in food processor. Spread batter into an 8-inch (20-cm) square baking dish. Refrigerate until batter thickens to a fudge-like consistency. Cut into squares.

Did You Know?

Carob pod, also called Saint John's Bread, has been consumed since ancient times; there are even references to it in the Bible. It is said that Saint John sustained himself for long periods on the nutrition found in carob fruit.

Health Facilitators	Nutrient Density Rating
Protein	High
Fat	Low
Carbohydrate	Very High
Enzymes	Very High
Antioxidants	Very High
Fiber	Very High

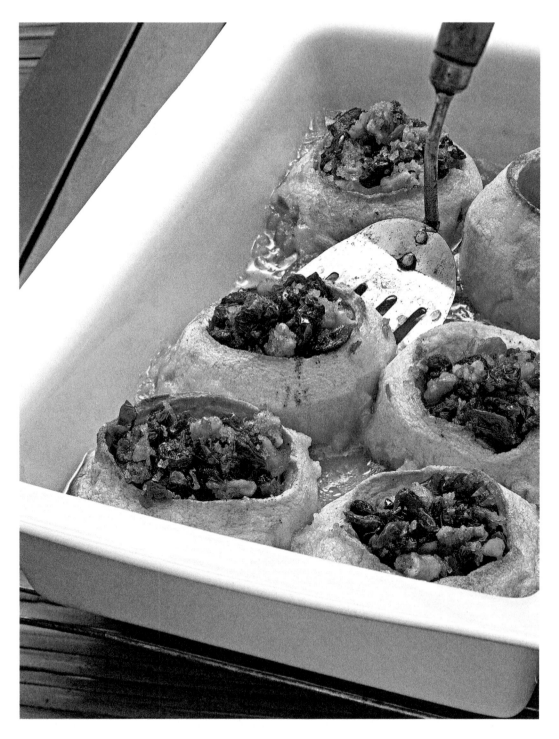

Baked Apples with Cherries and Walnuts

Apples are loaded with antioxidants and have numerous health benefits—they reduce the possibility of stroke, heart disease, wrinkles, and cancer, and they stimulate hair growth. Walnuts contain omega-3 essential fatty acids and contribute to brain function. Combine these with apples and cherries and you simply can't go wrong.

INGREDIENTS

6 large apples
6 tablespoons (85 g) unsalted butter, softened
½ cup (100 g) rapadura
2 tablespoons (28 ml) freshly squeezed lemon juice
⅓ cup (40 g) dried chopped cherries
3 tablespoons (24 g) chopped walnuts
1 tablespoon (5 g) grated lemon zest
1 teaspoon ground ginger
¼ teaspoon ground cloves

Yield: 6 servings

Health Facilitators	Nutrient Density Rating
Protein	High
Fat	Low
Carbohydrate	Moderate
Enzymes	Very High
Antioxidants	Very High
Fiber	Very High

Preheat oven to 350°F (180°C, or gas mark 4). Core apples from stem side through the center (but not all the way to bottom) and remove peels. Cream butter and rapadura. Stir in remaining ingredients, and place a spoonful of stuffing inside each apple. Place in a medium-size buttered baking pan with 2 to 3 tablespoons water. Bake for 1 hour, or until apples are tender.

Did You Know?

Cherries reduce inflammation, help with sleep, and prevent tooth decay. There is also evidence that cherries are so powerful they may reduce the risk of cancer by 50 percent. University of Iowa biochemist Raymond Hohl, M.D., found that cherries shut down the growth of cancer cells by depriving them of the proteins they need to grow.

Cherries also contain vitamins A and C, melatonin, and phytonutrients, such as bioflavonoids, anthocyanins, and ellagic acid, which help prevent damage to cells.

Thai-Style Bananas in Coconut Milk

Coconut stimulates metabolism and is therefore great for losing weight. Moreover, it has numerous health benefits: supporting your immune system; keeping your skin healthy and youthful looking; promoting heart health; and providing an immediate energy source. With a combination of coconut and bananas, a balanced food with loads of potassium, vitamins, minerals, and fiber, this dish delivers Mother Nature's perfect food and medicine.

INGREDIENTS
4 large ripe bananas
One 15-ounce (440-ml) can coconut milk
½ cup (100 g) coconut sugar
½ teaspoon Himalayan crystal salt
1 teaspoon pure vanilla extract
  or vanilla essence
2 tablespoons finely chopped fresh mint

Yield: 4 servings

Health Facilitators	Nutrient Density Rating
Protein	Moderate
Fat	Moderate
Carbohydrate	Very High
Enzymes	Moderate
Antioxidants	Very High
Fiber	Very High

Peel bananas, cut them in half lengthwise, and slice each half into 4 pieces crosswise. In a saucepan, heat coconut milk. Add coconut sugar, salt, and vanilla or vanilla essence. When mixture is hot and smooth, add bananas, and simmer for five minutes, or until bananas are cooked but retain their shape. Serve warm for best flavor. Garnish with fresh mint.

Did You Know?
Coconut sugar, used in many Thai and Indian dishes, is a coarse brown sugar with a distinct caramel flavor. It is not as sweet as cane sugar and contains a number of minerals and nutrients. Look for it online or in health food stores.

Zesty Strawberry-Rhubarb Pudding

Rhubarb is a perfect fruit for your fibromyalgia diet because it is high in calcium and inflammation-reducing antioxidants. Combined with delicious strawberries and a nice zest of lime, this pudding will have your taste buds feeling like they're in seventh heaven.

INGREDIENTS

5 cups (850 g) sliced organic strawberries, plus extra for garnish
2 cups (200 g) chopped rhubarb
1 teaspoon lemon zest
3 tablespoons (45 g) pure maple syrup
2 tablespoons (12 g) agar-agar flakes
1 tablespoon (6 g) kuzu, dissolved in 3 tablespoons (45 ml) filtered cold water
Fresh mint sprigs for garnish

Yield: 8 servings

In a medium saucepan, bring the strawberries, rhubarb, lemon zest, and maple syrup to a boil over medium-high heat. Sprinkle with the agar-agar flakes, reduce the heat to medium, and simmer until all the flakes are dissolved, about 10 minutes. Add the dissolved kuzu and stir until the mixture thickens. Transfer to a bowl or individual cups and refrigerate until set. Garnish with strawberry slices and a sprig of fresh mint.

Health Facilitators	Nutrient Density Rating
Protein	Low
Fat	Low
Carbohydrate	High
Enzymes	Moderate
Antioxidants	High
Fiber	High

Hearty Brown Rice Pudding

The high fiber content in brown rice is especially helpful in controlling cholesterol, which is of prime importance in preventing heart disease. Brown rice also contains vitamin B, vitamin E, antioxidants, and minerals. Toss in Mother Nature's perfect food—eggs—and a handful of high-energy pecans and raisins, which are loaded with phytochemicals, vitamin E, and fiber, and you have a dessert that's a powerhouse of nutritional benefits.

INGREDIENTS
3 eggs
1½ cups (355 ml) dairy or coconut cream
⅓ cup (110 g) maple syrup
1 teaspoon pure vanilla extract
⅛ teaspoon Himalayan crystal salt
½ teaspoon cinnamon
2 cups (380 g) cooked whole-grain
  brown rice
¾ cup (85 g) toasted pecans, chopped
2 cups (290 g) raisins
1 to 2 bananas, peeled and mashed
  (optional)

Yield: 8 to 10 servings

Preheat oven to 325°F (170°C, or gas mark 3). Beat eggs with cream, maple syrup, vanilla, salt, and cinnamon. Stir in rice, pecans, raisins, and bananas (if desired). Pour into a buttered casserole dish or soufflé dish. Bake for 50 minutes, or until pudding is just slightly loose in the center.

Did You Know?
Whole grains are believed to benefit the heart in a number of ways. The fiber and other nutrients in whole grains may help lower cholesterol, blood sugar, and insulin levels, as well as improve blood vessel functioning and reduce inflammation in the circulatory system.

Health Facilitators	Nutrient Density Rating
Protein	High
Fat	Moderate
Carbohydrate	Very High
Enzymes	Low
Antioxidants	High
Fiber	Very High

Fresh Fruit Salad Gone Nuts

There's nothing sweeter than the luscious flavors of fresh fruits in season. The colors of fresh berries blended together with apples, mango, papaya, or any other seasonal fruit is a sight for sore eyes and a wonderful pick-me-up at any time of the day or night. Go for any berry that you like because they are all loaded with antioxidants, especially vitamin C. They are also high in fiber, potassium, and iodine, which makes them great for boosting thyroid output. The addition of walnuts, which are high in omega-3 essential fatty acids, and the delicious balance of crème fraîche will stabilize your blood sugar levels as well. This dish makes a perfect snack, too.

INGREDIENTS
6 cups (900 g) chopped fresh seasonal fruits
¼ cup (45 g) pitted and chopped fresh dates
¼ cup (60 ml) freshly squeezed orange juice
1½ cups (345 g) crème fraîche or yogurt
3 tablespoons (24 g) chopped walnuts
6 fresh mint sprigs

Yield: 8 servings

Place the fruit in attractive serving bowls. In a mixing bowl, combine the chopped dates, orange juice, and crème fraîche and mix well. Place 3 tablespoons (45 g) of the creamy mixture on top of each serving of fruits and garnish with ½ tablespoon (4 g) of the chopped walnuts and a sprig of mint.

Health Facilitators	Nutrient Density Rating
Protein	Low
Fat	Low
Carbohydrate	Moderate
Enzymes	Moderate
Antioxidants	High
Fiber	High

Mmm... Chocolate Mousse

Chocolate stimulates the secretion of endorphins, which produce pleasurable sensations. It also contains potent antioxidant properties and the neurotransmitter serotonin, which acts as an anti-depressant. More good news: Chocolate provides us with several vitamins, including B1, B2, D, and E.

INGREDIENTS

6 large eggs, separated, at room temperature
2 tablespoons (28 ml) filtered water or strong coffee
1 teaspoon pure vanilla extract
4 tablespoons (50 g) sugar, divided
6 ounces (170 g) best-quality bittersweet chocolate, coarsely chopped
4 tablespoons (55 g) unsalted butter
¼ teaspoon cream of tartar

Yield: 6 servings

Health Facilitators	Nutrient Density Rating
Protein	Low
Fat	Very High
Carbohydrate	Moderate
Enzymes	Low
Antioxidants	High
Fiber	Low

Combine 4 egg yolks (you can discard the remaining two) in a medium heat-proof bowl with the water, vanilla extract, and 2 tablespoons (25 g) of sugar. Set the bowl on top of a small saucepan of simmering water. Whisk egg mixture until you begin to see the bottom of the bowl. Remove bowl from heat, immediately add the chocolate and butter, and whisk until smooth. If necessary, return the bowl to the saucepan of hot water to fully incorporate the ingredients.

Combine the 6 egg whites with cream of tartar in a mixing bowl. Beat with a whisk until whites are fluffy and have formed soft peaks, 4 to 7 minutes. Add remaining 2 tablespoons (25 g) of sugar and continue beating until whites are smooth and stiff peaks have formed, about 2 to 3 minutes.

Whisk about one-fourth of the beaten egg whites into the chocolate mixture, until the mixture is smooth and you see no traces of white. Pour this chocolate mixture over the remaining beaten egg whites and fold together. Scoop into a large serving bowl or into individual bowls or ramekins. Cover with plastic wrap, pushing the wrap down so that it touches the surface of the mousse (to avoid developing a "skin").

Refrigerate for at least 2 hours before serving.

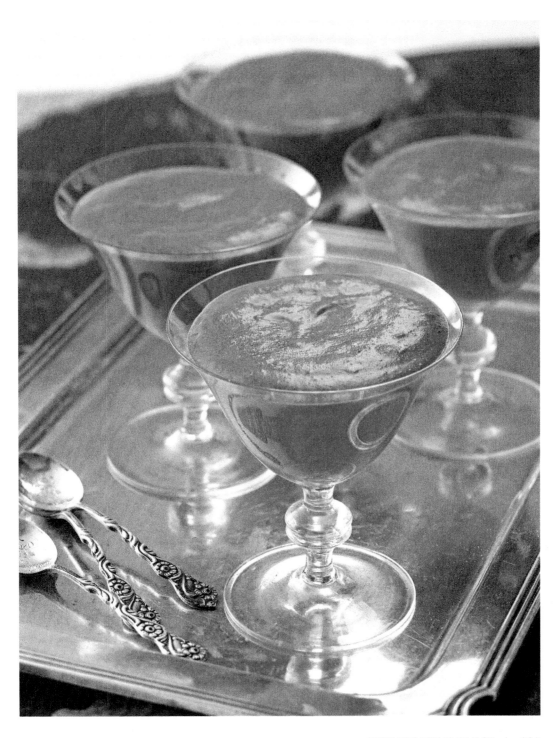

Apple Pie with Pizzazz (RAW)

This is an apple pie like no other. Walnuts are one of the best plant sources of protein, and they are rich in fiber, B vitamins, magnesium, and antioxidants such as vitamin E. Apples are loaded with antioxidants such as vitamin C, and they offer many health benefits. They also help in protecting against cancer, stroke, and heart disease and may play a role in slowing the aging process. Enjoy this pie for breakfast, as a snack, or as a dessert.

INGREDIENTS

1 cup (125 g) ground raw walnuts

1 cup (175 g) pitted dates, soaked in purified or spring water for 15 minutes and drained

½ cup (75 g) raw sunflower seeds, soaked in purified or spring water for 20 minutes, drained, and rinsed

1 cup (75 g) unsweetened shredded coconut, divided

4 cups (600 g) peeled, shredded apples

2½ teaspoons cinnamon

½ cup (120 ml) unfiltered apple juice

2/3 cup (110 g) raisins, dried figs, or prunes

Yield: 6 to 8 servings

Using a food processor, blend walnuts, dates, sunflower seeds, and 2/3 cup (50 g) of shredded coconut. Once mixture is smooth, press it into a 9-inch (23-cm) pie shell and set aside. Place grated apples in large mixing bowl. Blend together cinnamon, apple juice, and dried fruit, and spoon over grated apples. Mix thoroughly. Fill pie crust with apple filling and garnish it with remaining 1/3 cup (28 g) shredded coconut.

DID YOU KNOW?

Dates are an energy food known for their high levels of magnesium, calcium, and fiber.

Health Facilitators	Nutrient Density Rating
Protein	High
Fat	Low
Carbohydrate	Very High
Enzymes	Very High
Antioxidants	Very High
Fiber	Very High

All-Star Blueberry Cream Pie (RAW)

Blueberries are nutritional stars bursting with flavor and packed full of phytonutrients and antioxidants such as vitamins C and E. Their many benefits include warding off heart disease, improving nighttime vision, and protecting against all forms of cancer. Pecans are rich in antioxidants, magnesium, and fiber, and they are an excellent source of essential fatty acids.

INGREDIENTS

For crust

2 cups (200 g) pecans, soaked in purified or spring water overnight and drained

1 cup (165 g) raisins or dates, soaked in purified or spring water for 1 hour, drained, reserving 4 tablespoons (60 ml) of soaking water

1 tablespoon (14 g) cinnamon

For filling

4 cups (580 g) blueberries, divided

1½ cups (120 g) fresh coconut pulp, shredded

2 tablespoons (28 g) coconut butter or (28 ml) coconut oil

½ teaspoon cinnamon, plus dash for garnish

Yield: 6 to 8 servings

To make crust: Process all ingredients in a food processor until well combined. Press mixture into a 9-inch (23-cm) glass pie pan and dehydrate for 1 to 2 hours at 120°F (45°C).

To make filling: Process 2 cups (290 g) of blueberries, the coconut pulp, coconut butter or oil, and cinnamon in a blender until smooth. Pour filling into pie crust and chill for one hour before serving. Garnish with remaining 2 cups (290 g) of blueberries and dash of cinnamon.

DID YOU KNOW?

Coconuts contain lauric acid and its derivative, mono-laurin, which have properties that destroy viruses such as influenza. Coconuts are anti-inflammatory, anti-viral, anti-fungal, and anti-bacterial.

Health Facilitators	Nutrient Density Rating
Protein	Very High
Fat	Moderate
Carbohydrate	Very High
Enzymes	Very High
Antioxidants	Very High
Fiber	Very High

Rockin' Raspberry Sauce (RAW)

Plump, juicy raspberries are a summer favorite because of their naturally delicious and sweet flavor. Rich in vitamin C, folic acid, iron, and potassium, raspberries also provide high amounts of both insoluble fiber (thanks to those little seeds) and soluble fiber pectin. They are an excellent source of ellagic acid and many other disease-fighting antioxidants. To add protein and healthy omega-3s, serve the sauce with yogurt and walnuts or almonds.

INGREDIENTS

One 12-ounce (340-g) package
  frozen raspberries, partially thawed
½ cup (160 ml) maple syrup
1 to 2 cups (235 to 475 ml) pure water

Yield: 4 cups (950 ml)

Place raspberries in food processor with maple syrup, and process to make a thick paste. Gradually add water until desired consistency is reached.

Did You Know?

Raspberries contain a number of flavonoids called anthocyanins, which give the berries their rich red color. The anthocyanins also contain unique antioxidant properties, as well as some antimicrobial ones, including the ability to prevent the overgrowth of certain bacteria and fungi in the body, such as the yeast *Candida albicans*.

Health Facilitators	Nutrient Density Rating
Protein	None
Fat	None
Carbohydrate	High
Enzymes	High
Antioxidants	High
Fiber	High

Body-Building Banana Cherry Nut Bread

Creamy, rich, and sweet, bananas are a popular food with everyone from infants to elders. Bananas are one of our best sources of potassium, which is an essential mineral for maintaining normal blood pressure and heart function. Cherries are a rich source of melatonin and other potent antioxidants, such as vitamins A, C, and E.

INGREDIENTS

1⅓ cups (145 g) all purpose or
   gluten-free flour
1½ teaspoons baking powder
½ teaspoon baking soda
½ teaspoon Himalayan crystal salt
12 tablespoons (170 g) butter, softened
½ cup (100 g) rapadura or molasses (170 g)
2 eggs
⅓ cup (80 ml) skim milk
3 ripe bananas, mashed
¼ cup (40 g) dried cherries
2 tablespoons (15 g) chopped walnuts
1 tablespoon (15 ml) freshly squeezed
   lemon juice

Yield: 1 loaf

Preheat oven to 350°F (180°C, or gas mark 4). Lightly grease only the bottom of a 9- × 5-inch (23- × 13-cm) loaf pan. In a large mixing bowl, combine the flour, baking powder, baking soda, and salt. Set aside.

In another bowl, beat butter and rapadura (or molasses) until mixture is light and fluffy. Add eggs one at a time, beating well after each. Stir in milk, beating until well mixed. Add flour mixture, stirring into wet ingredients gradually, until just mixed.

Fold mashed bananas, cherries, walnuts, and lemon juice into batter. Scrape batter into loaf pan and bake for 40 to 45 minutes, or until toothpick inserted into center comes out clean. Let bread cool on rack for 10 minutes.

Loosen bread from sides of pan with a knife. Remove cake from pan and let it cool completely on rack.

Health Facilitators	Nutrient Density Rating
Protein	High
Fat	Moderate
Carbohydrate	Very High
Enzymes	Low
Antioxidants	Very High
Fiber	Very High

Did You Know?
Walnuts are an excellent source of protein and healthy fats, in addition to the essential fatty acids so beneficial for your immune system and in fighting inflammation.

Coconut Apple Nut Cake

There's something luscious about the combination of healthy-fat coconut; high-fiber, antioxidant-rich apples; and nuts. The natural sweetness of fruit in this delicious moist cake is nourishing as well as blood-sugar balancing and is sure to keep your energy levels in check. Its already delicious taste is heightened with the freshness of orange juice.

INGREDIENTS

4 large apples, cored, peeled, and sliced
2 tablespoons (15 g) chopped walnuts
4 teaspoons ground cinnamon
1 cup (145 g) raisins
6 fresh dates, pitted and chopped
2 cups (400 g) sugar
1 cup (120 g) coconut flour
1 tablespoon (14 g) baking powder
½ cup (120 ml) coconut oil
4 large eggs
½ cup (120 ml) freshly squeezed orange juice
1 tablespoon (14 g) butter, melted

Yield: One 10-inch (25-cm) cake

Preheat the oven to 350°F (180°C, or gas mark 4). Grease a 10-inch (25-cm) angel cake pan or spring-load pan. In a medium bowl, combine the apples, walnuts, cinnamon, raisins, and dates. In a separate bowl, combine the sugar, the flour, baking powder, oil, eggs, orange juice, and butter. With an electric mixer, beat for 4 to 5 minutes to make a smooth batter. Pour half the batter into the pan and spread half the apple mixture on top. Repeat with the remaining batter and apples and bake for 30 minutes. Then lower the oven temperature to 300°F (150°C, or gas mark 2) and bake for 1 hour longer, or until a toothpick inserted into the center comes out clean.

Health Facilitators	Nutrient Density Rating
Protein	Moderate
Fat	Low
Carbohydrate	High
Enzymes	Low
Antioxidants	Moderate
Fiber	High

Oatmeal Raisin Chews

Not your average cookie, these chewy raisin delights will become your go-to choice for comfort food that's close to your heart. They are full of fiber and goodness and so simple to make.

INGREDIENTS

2 cups (160 g) rolled oats
2 teaspoons ground cinnamon
2 teaspoons ground nutmeg
1 teaspoon ground coriander
¼ cup (20 g) shredded coconut
¼ cup (36 g) raisins
¼ cup (30 g) chopped walnuts or pecans
½ cup (120 ml) frozen concentrated apple juice
Dash of cayenne pepper (optional)
4 large egg whites
2 teaspoons molasses

Yield: 36 to 48 cookies

Preheat the oven to 375°F (190°C, or gas mark 5). Place the rolled oats on a baking sheet. Toast in the oven for 8 to 10 minutes, until lightly browned. Remove from the oven and place in a large mixing bowl. Add the cinnamon, nutmeg, coriander, coconut, raisins, nuts, apple juice, and cayenne and mix together. With an electric mixer, beat the egg whites until foamy. Beat in the molasses until stiff but not dry, then gently fold the egg whites into the oat mixture. Immediately drop the mixture by the teaspoon onto 2 nonstick cookie sheets and bake for 20 minutes, or until dark brown.

Health Facilitators	Nutrient Density Rating
Protein	Moderate
Fat	Low
Carbohydrate	High
Enzymes	Low
Antioxidants	Moderate
Fiber	High

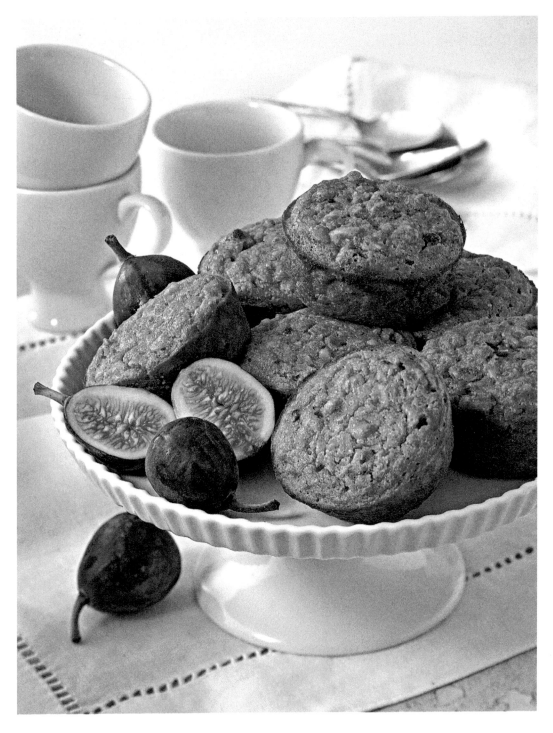

Digestive Orange and Fig Muffins

The nutritional value of figs closely resembles that of human milk—they are rich in vitamins A, B1, B2, and calcium, iron, phosphorus, manganese, sodium, and potassium. Figs are also high in fiber and help with intestinal regulation. Oranges have long been known as a rich source of vitamin C, as well as other phytonutrients, such as citrus limonoids compounds, which have been successful in fighting various types of cancer.

INGREDIENTS

6 large, fresh figs, peeled and finely chopped, or 1 to 1½ cups (150 to 225 g) dried and reconstituted figs, finely chopped
1 cup (125 g) plus 1 tablespoon (8 g) whole-wheat or gluten-free flour
1 cup (80 g) rolled oats
1 tablespoon (12 g) baking powder
½ teaspoon Himalayan crystal salt
3 teaspoons grated orange zest
1 teaspoon cinnamon
1 cup (235 ml) whole milk
2 eggs, lightly beaten
1/8 cup (40 g) molasses
8 tablespoons (112 g) butter, melted

Yield: 12 muffins

Preheat oven to 450°F (230°C, or gas mark 8). Grease 12 muffin cups. In a small bowl, toss chopped figs with 1 tablespoon (8 g) flour.

In a large bowl, mix 1 cup (125 g) flour, oats, baking powder, salt, orange zest, and cinnamon, and stir to combine well. In another large bowl, mix together milk, eggs, molasses, and melted butter. Gradually add dry ingredients to wet ingredients; fold in the figs.

Spoon batter into greased muffin cups, and bake for 10 to 15 minutes, or until toothpick inserted into center comes out clean.

Health Facilitators	Nutrient Density Rating
Protein	Moderate
Fat	Moderate
Carbohydrate	Very High
Enzymes	Low
Antioxidants	High
Fiber	Very High

Peanut Coconut Macaroons

Coconut is a highly nutritious food that's rich in lauric acid, a substance known for being anti-viral, antibacterial, and anti-fungal. It also makes your skin and hair lustrous and soft. Peanuts are a terrific plant source of protein, and they are rich in fiber, phytonutrients, and antioxidants, such as vitamin E and selenium. Go nuts with this pair of nutritious treats.

INGREDIENTS
4 egg whites
Pinch of salt
2½ cups (190 g) finely shredded coconut
½ cup (130 g) creamy peanut butter
⅓ cup (40 g) chopped peanuts

Yield: 15 to 20 macaroons

Health Facilitators	Nutrient Density Rating
Protein	Very High
Fat	Moderate
Carbohydrate	Moderate
Enzymes	Low
Antioxidants	Very High
Fiber	Very High

Preheat oven to 300°F (150°C, or gas mark 2). Line a baking sheet with buttered parchment paper. Beat egg whites with salt in a clean bowl until they form stiff peaks. Gradually fold in shredded coconut and peanut butter—you want to add enough so that the mixture will form balls but not so much that it becomes crumbly. Drop mixture by rounded teaspoons 2 inches (5 cm) apart onto baking sheets or shape them into balls, using fingertips. Sprinkle with chopped peanuts. Bake for 20 minutes. Reduce temperature to 200°F (93°C) and bake for 30 to 45 minutes for chewy macaroons; for crisp macaroons, bake for at least 1 hour. Remove from oven and cool completely before removing from parchment paper. Store in an airtight container.

No-Bake Almond Chocolate Oatmeal Cookies

Simple and delicious is the best way to describe these nutritious no-bake treats. Almonds are abundant in vitamin E, a heart-healthy nutrient, along with magnesium, fiber, and tryptophan, all of which make for an efficient metabolism. The combination of rolled oats and natural sweeteners will keep your blood sugar balanced, too.

INGREDIENTS

¼ cup (85 g) raw honey or molasses
½ cup (120 ml) brown rice syrup
3 cups (240 g) rolled oats
6 fresh dates, pitted and chopped
1 tablespoon (8 g) carob or cocoa
  powder
2 teaspoons vanilla extract
¼ cup (55 g) unsalted butter, melted
  (optional)
1 cup (260 g) almond butter
1 teaspoon ground cinnamon

Yield: 24 cookies

In a large bowl, combine the honey, syrup, oats, dates, carob powder, vanilla, butter, almond butter, and cinnamon. Form into cookie rounds, place on a large cookie sheet, and cover with waxed paper. Place in the refrigerator to set. Serve cold.

Health Facilitators	Nutrient Density Rating
Protein	Moderate
Fat	Low
Carbohydrate	High
Enzymes	Low
Antioxidants	Moderate
Fiber	High

CHAPTER 12

TONICS, TINCTURES, AND SUPERFOODS

In this chapter, I describe the types of natural food, vitamin, and mineral supplements recommended for use in dealing with the various disorders associated with fibromyalgia. Regaining optimum health and vitality depends upon a careful balance of at least fifty daily nutrients, whose sources include protein, carbohydrates, and fats. We have discussed the critical role of nutrition and choosing foods that nourish and strengthen you, in response to the evidence indicating that many of the nutritional deficiencies present with fibromyalgia are due to improper diet and eating habits. Because people with fibromyalgia tend to have digestion and absorption problems, and because the body's ability to absorb nutrients from food declines with age, there is a clear and compelling reason for taking supplements for nutritional support.

There are smaller requirements for some nutrients than others (for example, the requirement for selenium is less than a millionth of that for protein), but they are no less important. In fact, one-third of all chemical reactions in our bodies are dependent on tiny quantities of minerals, and even more reactions are dependent upon vitamins. One missing vitamin, mineral, or other nutrient will slow you

down, and without any of these nutrients, energy, vitality, and optimal functioning are simply not possible.

Natural food supplements come in several forms, including food-nutrients, tonics, and superfoods. Supplemental food-nutrients help the body combust food for use as energy. An example is the antioxidant vitamin C, which helps neutralize free radicals. Tonics, which contain concentrated extracts from beneficial herbs and plants, are used to help build up and tone the body systems. Tonics are generally made from nutritive and nourishing herbs, such as dandelion root and milk thistle, that are safe and beneficial as long-term energy aids. Superfoods are living, whole-food, green plant supplements, such as wheat grass and chlorella, known for their enzyme-loaded phytonutrients and concentrated levels of antioxidants, enzymes, vitamins, minerals, and amino acids. These nutrient supplements help to protect the body from free-radical damage and promote healing and new cell growth.

Before purchasing any nutritional supplement, be sure that the manufacturer has the scientific expertise to produce products that are safe and effective. In choosing nutrients and supplements, look for a manufacturer that follows GMP guidelines (Good Manufacturing Practice guidelines). These supplements are the highest standard available and ensure that manufacturing and quality control procedures have been carefully followed. You can generally find GMP certification standards noted on the product packaging. Furthermore, look for products that are free of fillers, binders, coloring agents, gluten, lactose, and sweeteners.

Let's take a detailed look at the most highly recommended nutrient supplements for people with fibromyalgia.

Energizing Nutrients

What you experience as energy—mental or physical—is the end result of a series of chemical reactions that take place in every cell in your body. Nutrients from food combust with oxygen to make a unit of cellular energy in the form of a chemical called adenosine triphosphate, or ATP, which in turn makes muscles work, nerve signals fire, and brain cells function. If we are missing vital nutrients, we are less able to extract energy from the food we eat. This results in low energy levels, weight gain, and food cravings.

Because fibromyalgia is akin to an energy crisis, we will focus on the nutrients that are vital to metabolism and that can energize your system from a cellular level. Here are a number of nutritional supplements that have proven especially beneficial in treating fibromyalgia.

D-Ribose (Corvalen)

D-ribose (Corvalen) is a nutrient that has been shown to play a highly beneficial adjunctive role in the metabolic treatment of fibromyalgia. It provides the structural foundation—the backbone, if you will—of the energy compound ATP. ATP is the primary source of energy for all living cells and is made from ribose. In tissues facing the metabolic stress of low oxygen, dysfunctional mitochondria, or poor energy metabolism—as is the in case with fibro-

myalgia—ATP is broken down, and the metabolic machinery used by the cell to recycle expended energy is disrupted. These reactions ultimately lead to increased concentrations of metabolic by-products that must be recycled or removed from the cell. Up to 90 percent of these metabolic by-products can be removed or salvaged, but if they are not recovered quickly, they are washed out of the cell and are lost forever. The loss of these by-products has the effect of draining the cell of energy and, over time, draining your whole body of energy.

In the cells, the process of salvaging energy by-products begins with D-ribose. In fact, the process cannot continue without ribose. As long as enough ribose is available, the process of energy salvage goes smoothly and quickly, but if ribose is not available in sufficient quantities, the process halts and energy is lost. Although the body makes ribose naturally, it does so slowly and cannot keep pace with the demand. Most tissues of the body lack the metabolic machinery to produce adequate amounts of ribose quickly. For this reason, when your body faces severe energy stress, supplementing with ribose helps keep energy in the cells and enables energy balance to be restored.

Ribose is also needed to make new energy compounds. The energy molecule ATP is made from ribose. Beginning with ribose, the body goes through a number of metabolic reactions to produce ATP. If there is not enough ribose in the cell, the process of making ATP cannot proceed. This explains why chronically stressed tissue and muscles, as in fibromyalgia, have such difficulty regaining an energy balance. Muscle cells cannot make ribose quickly, and the energy needs of muscle in fibromyalgia outpace the cell's ability to supply the energy it needs. Ribose supplementation helps the muscle speed the process of energy salvage and energy building, leading to a return of energy. Ribose supplementation provides the metabolic support the body needs to bypass the slow process of natural ribose production and stimulate the muscle's energy recovery.

Recently published studies have shown that after supplementing with D-ribose, fibromyalgia and chronic fatigue syndrome (CFS) sufferers enjoyed an average 44 percent increase in energy after only three weeks, and an average overall improvement in quality of life of 30 percent. Improvements were noted starting at twelve days, and two-thirds of the fibromyalgia and CFS patients felt they had improved. When you realize that a 10 percent improvement for a single nutrient is considered excellent, 44 percent is nothing short of amazing. Visit www.corvalen.com for more information pertaining to studies related to improvements in fibromyalgia using D-ribose.

Co-Enzyme Q10

Also known as Co-Q10, Co-Enzyme Q10 is a naturally occurring compound found in every cell in your body. It is critical in the production of energy within each cell. Without this energy, your cells cannot function. Co-Q10 is a substance needed for the proper functioning of an enzyme, a protein molecule that speeds up the rate at which chemical reactions take place in the body. Co-Q10 is also used by the body as an antioxidant, and it protects cells from free radicals. Co-Q10 can be found in high concentrations in tissues and organs that require a lot of energy. The heart requires huge amounts of energy to function, which is why Co-Q10 is important for proper heart function and crucial to maintaining cardiovascular health.

Digestive Enzymes

Digestive enzymes are important for normal digestion and are abundant in raw fruits and vegetables. After age 30 to 35, there is a decline in the level of digestive enzymes produced in the stomach, pancreas, and small intestine. These enzymes are beneficial for people with fibromyalgia because of their problems with digestion and nutrient absorption. Apart from promoting healthy digestion, digestive enzymes perform a variety of other necessary functions within the body, such as helping to reduce swelling and pain from inflammation and helping to speed up our recovery rate when the body is out of kilter or not in homeostasis (not in balance).

Trypsin and chymotrypsin, enzymes the body manufactures to digest protein, help prevent excessive blood clotting and platelet "stickiness" by dissolving blood clots and removing metabolic wastes. Enzymes have many uses, from treating autoimmune diseases to arthritis, chronic diseases, and, of course, fibromyalgia. It's only necessary to take digestive enzyme supplements when eating cooked or processed foods, because raw (living) foods retain their enzymes.

Vitamins, Minerals, and Supplements

An integral part of any fibromyalgia diet are vitamin and mineral supplements. Certain daily supplements are recommended as part of a natural preventive program and are an important element of fibromyalgia self care, because they can help to alleviate a variety of fibromyalgia symptoms. Vitamins are not only an essential component to any healthy diet but are needed for basic biological processes, such as growth, nerve function, and digestion.

Minerals are the building blocks for enzymes and also help to regulate fluid in the body and control nerve movement. Any decision you make to take supplements as part of your wellness plan should be determined in conjunction with a knowledgeable practitioner.

Vitamin E

This vitamin is a powerful antioxidant that protects cells in the body from damage caused by free radicals. It is especially important in protecting blood cells, the nervous system, skeletal muscle, and the retinas in the eye from free-radical damage. Studies show that vitamin E also contributes to a healthy circulatory system, aids in proper blood clotting, and improves wound healing. The amount of vitamin E you need will vary according to your age, gender, and overall health. Also, your supplementary requirement will be less if your diet is naturally high in foods containing vitamin E, such as wheat germ, avocado, vegetable oil, egg yolks, nuts, and liver.

Vitamin C

An essential antioxidant that has many functions in the body, vitamin C aids in wound healing, prevents periodontal disease, enhances absorption of dietary iron, and maintains the body's collagen and connective tissue, which helps strengthen blood flow to vital organs such as the brain and heart. The Centers for Disease Control and Prevention estimate that people with high blood levels of vitamin C live six years longer than those with lower levels. Many people are deficient in vitamin C, particularly if they smoke, drink alcohol, or are taking antibiotics, cortisone, aspirin, or other pain medications. Additionally, deficiencies can result from exposure to toxic chemicals, from taking birth control pills, or because you are older than 60 years of age.

B-Complex

B-complex includes eight water-soluble vitamins that play important roles in cell metabolism. The eight vitamins are thiamine (B1), riboflavin (B2), niacin (B3), pyridoxine (B6), cobalamine (B12), folic acid, pantothenic acid, and biotin. The other related substances include choline, inositol, and para-amino benzoic acid (PABA). Although each vitamin or related substance performs a different function in the body, they all work together to maintain good health and vitality. A well-balanced diet should provide all the required B vitamins, but, because they are water soluble and therefore not retained by the body, we need a daily dietary supply. These vitamins are crucial for supporting the nervous system, the metabolism of protein, fat, and carbohydrate, and for energy production within the body.

5-Hydroxytryptophan (5-HTP)

Hydroxytryptophan (5-HTP) is an amino acid that is the intermediate step between tryptophan and the important neurotransmitter, serotonin. 5-HTP is proving effective in the treatment of fibromyalgia because the disorder is linked to a deficiency of serotonin. In a double-blind study, fifty patients with fibromyalgia were given either 100 milligrams of 5-HTP or a placebo three times per day. The group receiving the 5-HTP experienced significant improvements in their symptoms. In contrast, the group that received the placebo did not improve much at all. Improvements were noted across all symptom categories: number of painful areas; morning stiffness; sleep patterns; anxiety; and fatigue. Although 5-HTP tends to yield very good results within thirty days, even better results are obtained at ninety days.

Magnesium

Magnesium is critical to many cellular functions, including energy production, protein formation, and cellular replication. Magnesium participates in more than 300 enzymatic reactions in the body, particularly those processes that produce energy (for example, the production of ATP). When magnesium levels are low, energy levels are low. Because low magnesium levels are a common finding in patients with fibromyalgia, magnesium supplementation as part of treatment has produced very good results. Take magnesium bound to citrate, malate, fumarate, succinate, or aspartate—these are the forms that your body can most readily absorb and use.

Probiotics

Live microorganisms that support a healthy digestive system, probiotics maintain a balance between the harmful and beneficial bacteria in the gut. Illness, poor diet, stress, aging, infection by food poisoning, and the use of medications can upset the balance of beneficial to harmful bacteria. Probiotics are especially helpful when taken during and after antibiotic treatment, or when traveling abroad to places in which the body is likely to encounter different types of bacteria than those to which it is accustomed. Studies found that probiotics may improve nutrient bioavailability—available for the body to use and assimilate—including B vitamins, calcium, iron, zinc, copper, magnesium, and phosphorus.

Omega-3 Essential Fatty Acids

These include eicosapentaenoic acid (EPA) and docosahexaenoic acid (DHA). Both are found primarily in cold-water fish, such as salmon, herring, mackerel, and sardines. Other than fresh seaweed, plant foods rarely contain EPA or DHA. However, a third omega-3 called alpha-linolenic acid (ALA) is found primarily in dark green leafy vegetables, flaxseed oils, and certain vegetable oils. The body can convert alpha-linolenic acid into EPA and DHA. Omega-3s have anti-inflammatory properties. They have been shown to improve rheumatoid arthritis, lupus, Raynaud's disease, and other autoimmune diseases. This is probably because the omega-3 fatty acids help the arteries, as well as many other parts of the body, stay inflammation-free. Other health benefits of omega-3s include alleviating depression, reducing LDL cholesterol levels and hypertension, and helping to prevent cancer.

Tonics

Tonic herbs strengthen and improve specific organs, systems, weaknesses, and the body as a whole. They are used to stimulate and optimize the function of organs that are not operating at their highest level or potential.

St. John's Wort (*Hypericum perforatum*)

St. John's Wort is known for its ability to relieve mild depression and improve sleep quality, both of which are typically present with fibromyalgia. It can be taken in tincture or extract form for concentrated potency levels.

Milk Thistle (*Silybum marianum*)

Milk thistle has been used medicinally for more than 2,000 years, most commonly in healing the liver and gallbladder. It contains a flavonoid called silymarin, an antioxidant that protects liver cells from toxins. (The terms "milk thistle" and "silymarin" are often used interchangeably.) Silymarin's anti-inflammatory effects keep liver cells from swelling in response to injury. Silymarin promotes liver-cell protein synthesis and decreases the oxidation of glutathione (a potent antioxidant). It can be taken in tincture or extract form for concentrated potency levels.

Dandelion (*Taraxacum officinale*)

Dandelion leaves and roots are a good source of iron, potassium, sodium, and calcium and have been used for centuries to treat liver, gall bladder, kidney, and joint problems. The leaves are a richer source of vitamin A than carrots, and they contain vitamins B, C, and D. Dandelion is also useful as a blood purifier and is helpful in treating disorders such as eczema and cancer. It has also been used to improve poor digestion, relieve water retention, and treat diseases of the liver, such as hepatitis. It is a good tonic for people with fibromyalgia; by helping the liver, it works to purify the whole system. It can be combined in tincture or extract form with St. John's wort.

Ginkgo Biloba

Used by the Chinese for almost 2,800 years as a natural medicine and tonic to treat a variety of conditions, ginkgo biloba contains numerous antioxidants, such as flavonoids, to counteract free radicals. Flavonoids are known to strengthen capillaries, thereby easing blood flow to the brain, helping to maintain cognitive health, and improving memory. Ginkgo works as a blood thinner to increase blood flow and reduce plaque. Ginkgo also increases metabolism efficiency and boosts oxygen levels, particularly in the brain, which uses 20 percent of the body's total supply of oxygen.

Superfoods

Used by certain traditional peoples in Latin America, Africa, and elsewhere for millennia, green superfoods, such as blue-green algae, chlorella, spirulina, and cereal grasses such as barley and wheat, are an important category of phytonutrient-rich nutritional products. These green foods naturally contain high concentrations of chlorophyll and are harvested seasonally to take advantage of enzymes and high potencies of naturally occurring nutrients. Some forms of micro-algae are thought to contain every nutrient required by the human body, although certain nutrients are present only in minute quantities. Superfoods are alkaline and help promote a healthy pH in your body.

Blue-Green Algae, Chlorella, and Spirulina

Blue-green algae, chlorella, and spirulina are the richest whole-food sources of protein, pro-vitamin A, and chlorophyll. Chlorophyll is the green pigment in plants that harnesses the sun's energy in photosynthesis. It is to plants what blood is to humans and is essential to metabolic functions, such as respiration and growth. In fact, the chlorophyll molecule is chemically similar to human blood, except that its central atom is magnesium whereas that of human blood is iron. It is used to repair tissues and helps neutralize pollutants in the food we eat and in the air we breathe, and it works to strengthen and purify the entire body. Chlorophyll has anti-inflammatory properties useful in treating fibromyalgia (as well as rheumatic and arthritis conditions), and it helps in the renewal of the liver and the blood. Green leafy vegetables, such as kale, collards, and parsley, are full of chlorophyll.

Chlorella is believed to contain the most chlorophyll of any plant. It also contains protein (about 58 percent), carbohydrates, fiber, amino acids, fatty acids, carotenoids, and numerous vitamins and minerals, including all of the B, C, and E vitamins. Chlorella stimulates the production of interferon, which helps your body's immune system. It helps to rejuvenate and revitalize the entire body by maintaining and repairing cells, stimulating growth of new cells, and supporting immune-system function. It's highly beneficial for fibromyalgia patients because of its nutrient density and the energy it provides. The chlorophyll in chlorella is very high in RNA and DNA, and it serves to cleanse the bloodstream. It generally comes in small tablets that can be crushed to break open its hard cell walls, allowing better assimilation of nutrients inside the body.

Spirulina, like chlorella, is well known for its chlorophyll and protein content, in addition to its high concentrations of vitamins, minerals, and amino acids. Spirulina is a naturally digestible food that aids in mineral absorption. It supplies nutrients needed to help cleanse the liver and heal, while curbing the appetite, making it beneficial for those who are fasting or have hypoglycemia. It is known for its immune-boosting capacity and its ability to bolster natural killer-cell function. Natural killer cells, a chief component of the immune system, play a major role in the rejection of tumors and virally infected cells. Spirulina is a nourishing food that's highly beneficial for anyone with fibromyalgia.

Wheat Grass and Barley Grass

Like micro-algae , wheat grass and barley grass contain high levels of chlorophyll and vitamin A and are rich sources of concentrated nutrients that have proven beneficial in treating fibromyalgia. Wheat grass and barley grass have almost identical therapeutic properties, although the latter may digest more easily. People with allergies to wheat generally have no allergic reactions to these superfoods. In their dried state, both of these grasses rank behind micro-algae in chlorophyll and vitamin A. Cereal grasses possess anti-inflammatory properties and have been especially helpful in treating fibromyalgia, as well as arthritis and rheumatism.

SUGGESTED READING

Books

A Consumer's Dictionary of Food Additives
By Ruth Winter, M.S.

This valuable reference provides all the facts about the relative safety and side effects of more than 12,000 ingredients—including preservatives, food-tainting pesticides, and animal drugs—that end up in your food as a result of processing and curing.

Beyond Antibiotics: 50 (or so) Ways to Boost Immunity and Avoid Antibiotics
By Michael A. Schmidt, Lendon H. Smith, and Keith W. Sehnert

Doctors fear that if antibiotic use is not curtailed, we may soon approach the day when untreatable infections are rampant. In *Beyond Antibiotics*, Schmidt, Smith, and Sehnert explore the problems presented by the overuse of antibiotic drugs. More importantly, they show how to build immunity, improve resistance to infections, and avoid antibiotics when possible.

Digestive Wellness
By Elizabeth Lipski, Ph.D., M.S., C.C.N.

Written by noted nutritionist Elizabeth Lipski, this popular resource provides the latest information and research on digestive disorders and is designed to help you understand the complex relationships between gastrointestinal physiology, diet, and health.

Dr. Mercola's Total Health Program
By Joseph Mercola, M.D.

This book is built entirely around a natural approach to diet and eating, including eating only the cleanest and healthiest forms of proteins, fats, and carbohydrates. The book addresses a range of subjects, including building your body's immune system to its peak level to help prevent or heal common illnesses; boosting your energy and mental clarity; attaining your body's optimal weight while still being satisfied and enjoying what you eat; helping to eliminate the underlying causes for those currently challenged by diseases and conditions such as chronic fatigue, allergies, heart problems, and diabetes.

Drug-Induced Nutrient Depletion Handbook
By Ross Pelton, R.Ph., Ph.D., C.N.N., James B. LaValle, R.Ph., D.H.M., N.M.D., C.C.N., and Earnest B. Hawkins, R.Ph., and Daniel L. Krinsky R.Ph., M.S.

Written by a team of pharmacists, this book is the most comprehensive book on the topic of how drugs affect nutrition.

Excitotoxins: The Taste That Kills
By Russell L. Blaylock, M.D.

Excitotoxins are substances added to foods and beverages that literally stimulate neurons to death, causing varying degrees of brain damage. Excitotoxins can be found in such ingredients as monosodium glutamate, aspartame, Cysteine, hydrolyzed protein, and aspartic acid. This book provides a detailed and well-researched look at the hazardous relationships of certain "foods" and brain health.

Fast Food Nation
By Eric Schlosser

This book provides a revealing, "behind the scenes" look at what goes into our nation's fast food industry.

Food Additives: A Shopper's Guide to What's Safe and What's Not, D.C.
By Christine Hoza Farlow

This pocket-sized book can be used conveniently in the supermarket to serve as a guide for the food additives found in many foods.

Food and Behavior: A Natural Connection
By Barbara Reed Stitt

Nutritionist Barbara Stitt focuses on how food allergies, and hypoglycemia, can adversely affect our behavior. As a probation officer, Stitt was able to help some of her parolees reform by changing their diets. She was amazed at the way in which personalities changed as food allergens were deleted from their diets.

From Fatigued to Fantastic, Third Edition
By Jacob Teitelbaum, M.D.

Written by renowned internist Jacob Teitelbaum, whose own medical education was interrupted by a bout of chronic fatigue syndrome and fibromyalgia, Teitelbaum has made these disorders his specialty. The book contains a wealth of information on these ailments, and the recommendations encompass dietary modifications, vitamin and mineral supplements, acupuncture, massage, chiropractic treatment, herbs, simple home remedies, and psychotherapy.

Health and Nutrition Secrets That Can Save Your Life
By Russell L. Blaylock, M.D.

This book, by Russell L. Blaylock, a certified neurosurgeon and clinical assistant professor of neurosurgery at the Medical University of Mississippi, is a 459-page holistic instruction manual and guide for improving personal health and avoiding common toxins and other environmental health hazards.

Living in Balance: A Dynamic Approach for Creating Harmony & Wholeness in a Chaotic World
By Joel Levey and Michelle Levey

This book is grounded in suggestions for finding harmony in love, work, eating, sleeping, exercise, and even breathing. The authors teach readers how to stay calm and balanced in their own "perfectly balanced oceans," regardless of the storms at sea.

Quantum Healing: Exploring the Frontiers of Mind/Body Medicine
By Deepak Chopra, M.D.

Chopra, a respected endocrinologist, brings together the current research of Western medicine, neuroscience, and physics with the insights of Ayurvedic theory in Quantum Healing to show that the human body is controlled by a "network of intelligence" grounded in quantum reality. He believes that intelligence exists everywhere in our bodies, in each of our 50 trillion cells, and that each cell knows how to heal itself. Through this intelligence lies the ability to change the basic patterns that design physiology, with the potential to defeat cancer, heart disease, and even aging itself.

Staying Healthy with Nutrition, 21st Century Edition: Complete Guide to Diet & Nutritional Medicine
By Elson M. Haas, M.D. with Buck Levin, Ph.D.

This book provides a thorough and intensive discussion of nutritional medicine and compiles decades of practical experience and scientific research into one encyclopedic volume. Building a healthy diet, the building blocks of nutrition, herbal supplements, homeopathic medicines, environmental aspects of nutrition, and detoxification and healing programs are just a few of the subjects discussed at length in this book.

Sugar Shock! How Sweets and Simple Carbs Can Derail Your Life–How You Can Get it Back on Track
By Connie Bennett, C.H.H.C. with Stephen T. Sinatra, M.D.

A well-written book on the deleterious effects of sugar on the body, based on the insights of thousands of physicians, nutritionists, researchers, and "sugar sufferers" worldwide. The book not only discusses the harmful effects of sugar on the body, it offers advice on how everyone can kick the sugar habit.

The 20-Day Rejuvenation Diet Program
By Jeffrey S. Bland, Ph.D., Ph.D. with Sarah Denum, M.A.

A well-researched reference book that explains the human body, the digestion process, and the detoxifying properties of the liver, as well as how to help the liver and your entire organism be healthier. It analyzes the foods that are and are not healthy for the body and how they relate to its function. Devising your own eating style is recommended, because each person is biochemically unique, and this book acknowledges this.

The Crazy Makers: How the Food Industry Is Destroying Our Brains and Harming Our Children
By Carol N. Simontacchi

A certified clinical nutritionist, Simontacchi explains how the food industries, which give us packaged, processed, and artificially flavored and colored foods, are destroying our bodies and our brains, all in the name of profit.

Your Body's Many Cries for Water
By F. Batmanghelidj, M.D.

Asthma, allergies, arthritis, hypertension, depression, headaches, diabetes, obesity, and MS: these are just some of the conditions and diseases that are caused by persistent dehydration, according to the research done by Dr. Fereydoon Batmanghelidj. But there is a miracle solution that is readily available, all natural, and free: water. In this book, Batmanghelidj reveals how easy it is to obtain optimum health by drinking more water and supports his claims with more than twenty years of clinical and scientific research.

Articles

"A Medical Food-Supplemented Detoxification Program in the Management of Chronic Health Problems," *Alternative Therapy*, J.S. Bland, E. Barrager. R.G. Reedy, K. Bland, 1995

"Chronic Fatigue Syndrome: Oxidative Stress and Dietary Modifications," *Alternative Medicine Review*, A.C. Logan, N.D. and C. Wong, N.D. 2001

"Fibromyalgia and Chronic Fatigue," *Heart, Health & Nutrition*, Stephen Sinatra, M.D., July 2007

"Nutritional Genomics: The Next Frontier in the Post Genomic Era," Physiological Genomics, J. Kaput and R.L. Rodriguez, 2003

ACKNOWLEDGMENTS

It's difficult to adequately acknowledge and thank the scores of people who contributed to the development of this book.

Like many people involved in nutritional research, I'm very grateful for the scientific legacy of great innovators such as Weston Price, D.D.S.; Francis Pottenger, M.D.; Emanuel Cheraskin, M.D., D.M.D.; Peter D'Adamo, N.D.; James D'Adamo, N.D.; Royal Lee, D.D.S.; George Watson, Ph.D.; Deepak Chopra, M.D.; David Hawkins, M.D., Ph.D.; and William Crook, M.D., to name only a few.

Very special thanks go to Rudolph Ballentine, M.D.; Abram Hoffer, M.D., Ph.D.; Morton Walker, D.P.M.; Bernard Jensen, D.C.; Carl C. Pfeiffer, M.D., Ph.D.; Samuel Epstein, M.D.; Candace B. Pert, Ph.D.; Andrew Weil, M.D.; Gabriel Cousens, M.D.; Sherry Rogers, M.D.; Doris Rapp, M.D.; Ann Louise Gittleman, Ph.D.; and Jeffrey Bland, Ph.D.

My heartfelt appreciation and thanks goes to Tom Vonderbrink and to Jim Herrick from Bioenergy Life Science, Inc. for believing and trusting in me and whose support contributed to the creation of this book.

I am very grateful for the support and keen insights of Jill Alexander and Amanda Waddell at Fair Winds Press, and to the fine editorial team including Nancy King, Pat Price, and Kathy Dragolich. Thanks also to: Ed Claflin, my agent; Catrine Kelty, food stylist, who did such an excellent job cooking and preparing the recipes; Glenn Scott for his talented photography; and Rosalind Wanke, Daria Perreault, and Visible Logic for the design of the book.

Jacob Teitelbaum, M.D. deserves very special thanks for his vital contributions to the research and development of using balanced nutrition principles and vitamin and mineral supplements to make fibromyalgia and chronic fatigue syndrome treatable and beatable conditions.

Above all, I'd like to thank my husband, Jonathan, whose remarkable talents, wisdom, and dedication have made so much possible, and who continues to be an inspiration.

Finally, I am eternally grateful to all the researchers, physicians, and scientists who over the years have strived to better understand the use of natural medicines. Without their work, this book could not have been written.

ABOUT THE AUTHOR

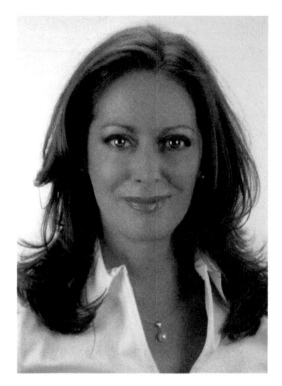

For more than a decade Deirdre Rawlings, N.D., Ph.D., has helped clients to overcome pain and fatigue, increase their energy, and attain optimum levels of health and wellness using the healing powers of food and nutrition. Deirdre's passion for functional nutrition was ignited by her success in healing her own fatigue, food allergies, digestive issues, hormone imbalances, and immune system disorders.

Deirdre is traditional naturopath, certified nutritionist, sports nutritionist, master herbalist, and certified health and wellness coach. She holds a Ph.D. in holistic nutrition, a master's in holistic nutrition, a master's in herbal medicine, and is board certified by the American Naturopathic Medical Certification Board, and Wellcoaches ®.

Deirdre practices clinical nutrition, using her knowledge of biochemistry, nutrition, herbs, functional medicine, and the power of the mind to return the body to a state of natural, vibrant health. She specializes in fibromyalgia, chronic fatigue syndrome, digestive disturbances, food allergies, and hormone balancing. Her online health and wellness courses and coaching programs have empowered thousands of people around the globe to remove the obstacles to optimum health, access their inner healer, and take charge of their own health.

Visit her websites at www. FoodsforFibromyalgia.com and www.RelaxationYogaNidra.com

INDEX

CPSIA information can be obtained at www.ICGtesting.com
Printed in the USA
LVOW05s0947180515

438614LV00005B/5/P